GOOD HOUSEKEEPING
EATING FOR A HEALTHY SKIN

GW00500559

Good Housekeeping Eating for a Healthy Skin

Alix Kirsta

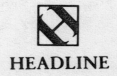

HEADLINE

Introduction copyright © 1989 Alix Kirsta
Recipes copyright © 1989 The National Magazine Company Ltd

First published in Great Britain in 1989
by Ebury Press,
an imprint of Century-Hutchinson Ltd

First published in this edition in 1990
by HEADLINE BOOK PUBLISHING PLC

10 9 8 7 6 5 4 3 2 1

ISBN 0 7472 3281 4

Typeset by Colset Private Limited, Singapore

Printed and bound in Great Britain by Collins, Glasgow

HEADLINE BOOK PUBLISHING PLC
Headline House, 79 Great Titchfield Street, London W1P 7FN

Contents

Introduction   1
A–Z of Skin Problems   59
Recipe Analysis and Nutrition Labelling   73
 1 Breakfast and Brunch   75
 2 Soups   89
 3 Starters   99
 4 Light Meals and Snacks   109
 5 Fish Main Dishes   125
 6 Meat and Poultry Main Dishes   141
 7 Vegetarian Main Dishes   157
 8 Vegetable Accompaniments   173
 9 Seasonal Salads   183
10 Barbecue Dishes   199
11 Puddings and Desserts   209
12 Baking   223
Index   239

Introduction

If there is any truth in the adage that 'we are what we eat', then the condition of our skin surely offers the most visible reflection of the benefits of healthy eating or the ill effects of an unbalanced diet. Contrary to popular belief, 'good' skin, in many cases, is not born to us but is either 'made', while poor skin is at least vastly improved through early recognition that true beauty can never be merely skin deep. Far from it. The human skin, its upsets, idiosyncrasies, characteristic patina, tone and texture, together represent the best possible advertisement for inner wellbeing – or the absence of it. It would indeed take a perverse quirk of nature to prevent the skin (and also, to a certain degree, the nails and hair) from giving away the state of our inner health. The relationship between the outer and inner body, though not immediately obvious, is intimate in the extreme. In order to carry out its many complex functions, let alone present an aesthetically appealing front to the outside world, skin tissue is crucially dependent on the synchronized mechanism of virtually all other internal organs and systems, whose balanced function is, in turn, largely determined by the quality of the daily diet.

The best examples of how skin responds as a sensor to physical, as well as psychological, change, can be observed, sometimes to quite dramatic effect, at times of stress, illness, or major hormonal transition, such as puberty, pregnancy or the menopause. All of these physical states represent periods of often very major biological flux or upheaval and may be accompanied by nutritional deficiencies or imbalances resulting in the need for an adjustment in diet. The visible improvement in many skin ailments, which so often occurs as a result of a change or modification of regular eating habits, offers living proof of the degree to which the quality and range of our regular diet both directly and indirectly influence the overall condition of the skin.

Impeccable hygiene, proper cleansing, the use of moisturizing creams and special protective or therapeutic skin oils and ointments, are all stratagems with an undeniably useful part to play in helping skin to remain good looking and youthful, and in protecting it against the ravages of external elements, such as harsh winds, extreme temperatures, pollution, and, above all, sunlight. But that is only a part of the picture. To be fully effective, really in-depth skincare cannot exist in isolation from more generalized health care. The two are intimately linked and interdependent and both ideally share an underlying holistic philosophy in which mind, emotions, body, nutrition, lifestyle and environment are recognized as contributory factors in our total, individual wellbeing. However, as I have tried to indicate in this book, it is nutrition, and the myriad elements that constitute healthy, balanced eating, which provides the most fascinating, if complex, set of clues to the puzzle of skin and its numerous diverse ailments and chronic disorders.

Although there may be many mysteries yet to be unravelled and riddles to be solved regarding this most paradoxical and important part of the human body, it is certain that no exploratory voyage into its interior is possible without background knowledge of the principles of healthy eating. In discovering how and why the foods we eat play such an important role in the condition of skin, it is important not to overlook the fact that the benefits gained, as we shall see, inevitably go far deeper than the outer surface.

SKIN STRUCTURE AND FUNCTION

No other visible part of the body records the shifting patterns of health as accurately as the skin. Far from being merely a pretty surface, an inert outer wrapping designed to protect and cushion internal organs and fluid from external damage, skin in fact qualifies as the largest, most complex and hardworking organ of the human body. Not only is its own function directly dependent on that of other organs and major systems, for example the liver and kidneys, the nervous system, hormone production and the circulation of blood and lymph fluids, but the skin itself represents a key element in the workings of general body chemistry. For example, along with the lungs, kidney and liver, the skin has a major part to play in the process of elimination, excreting up to 2 litres (3½ pints) of fluid every day, about 20 per cent of the body's total fluid loss.

Therein lies the supreme paradox of skin: 20 per cent fluid, accounting for somewhere between 2.7 and 3.6 kg (6 and 8 lb) total weight, its surface area measuring on average 1.6 square metres (17 square feet), skin tissue comprises a myriad network of nerve cells, blood vessels, sweat and sebaceous glands, hair follicles, pores and muscle fibre, all densely packed together and working round the clock to help regulate body temperature, excrete waste matter, counteract infection and convey a multitude of different sensations. As a self-propagating organ with about 20,000,000 cells packed into every square inch of tissue, healthy skin is constantly repairing and renewing itself, with cell division most prolific between the hours of midnight and 4 a.m.

THE EPIDERMIS

The dynamics of production never cease. An analysis of a cross section of skin tissue reveals a tidy pattern of cause and effect. The epidermis, the outer visible part of the skin, also known as the stratum corneum or keratin layer, is made up of the same tough protein substance that forms the hair and nails.

KERATINIZATION
This keratin layer is constantly being sloughed off and replaced by the upward migration of living basal cells, actively dividing lower down at the base of the epidermis. The day-to-day appearance of facial and body skin depends very largely on the prompt regular turnover of fresh cells at this basal level.

The process of co-called 'keratinization' represents the outermost manifestation of skin health and beauty. Any slowing down or, indeed, rapid and unnatural acceleration of keratinization can result in any number of skin disorders ranging from excessive dryness, dullness and premature ageing to more serious complaints, such as psoriasis. As with most other bodily functions, skin renewal begins to slow down gradually from the age of 35 or 40, becoming more markedly slow in the fifties and sixties.

MELANIN
Pigment cells, or 'melanocytes', responsible for manufacturing melanin, which gives the skin its basic colour and causes white skin to tan when exposed to the sun, are also scattered amongst the basal cells within the lower epidermis. The number and distribution of these melanocytes, as well as their ability to produce pigment in sunlight, is entirely genetically determined.

ANTIGEN-PRESENTING (AP) CELLS
Also situated within the epidermis are so-called 'langerhans cells' and 'Granstein cells', collectively termed 'antigen presenting' (AP) cells. Through their ability to monitor foreign substances and transmit messages to the white blood cells, telling them to produce T-helper and T-suppressor cells, the AP cells are believed to play an important role in the body's immune system.

THE DERMIS

Beneath the epidermis lies the 'true skin', the dermis, 1.8 mm (1/6 inch) thick and the centre of all skin life. Basically a fibrous protein mass, the dermis (also known as the connective tissue) is made up of a complex weave of collagen and other protein fibres embedded in a gel-like substance which helps nourish and bind water to the tissues and fibroblast cells responsible for manufacturing collagen. It is here that any sign of organic illness, hormonal imbalance, nutritional deficiency or faulty circulation first registers.

THE DERMIS AT WORK

Blood vessels, components of the lymphatic system, nerve endings, oil and sweat glands, with ducts and follicles leading to the surface, are all situated in the dermis where the skin joins forces with other body systems. An intricate network of tiny capillaries brings fresh oxygen and nutrients to the cells of the dermis, wastes are eliminated and dispersed via lymph and blood, and the sebaceous glands manufacture sebum which helps to lubricate the skin. Ageing, illness, excessive dehydration due to environmental factors, or eating an unbalanced diet, are the principal causes of insufficient lubrication which, in turn, leads to dryness, scaling and surface wrinkling.

Here too is located the body's central thermostat. As body temperature rises, the sweat glands counteract the effect by allowing extra moisture to evaporate via the pores, while fresh supplies of blood course to the skin's surface to aid the cooling-off process. (About one-third of fresh blood pumped from the heart is contained in the skin and 85 per cent of body heat is lost via the skin.)

The skin's blood vessels follow a loop-like circuit made up of arteries that supply blood, rich in oxygen and nutrients, and veins that carry away waste matter. The arteries, which eventually branch out into a vast and dense fretwork of arterioles and capillaries, assist the passage of oxygen, water, proteins, fats and carbohydrates from the blood into the tissues. Waste products travel in the opposite direction via the lymph system and along a network of bigger veins which carry toxins away from the tissues back to the circulation, where they are excreted via the kidneys and lungs.

All sensation, including differences of hot and cold, pleasure and pain, are recorded through the millions of nerve fibres, also clustered within the dermis and lower epidermis. Beneath the dermis, within the subcutaneous tissue, or hypodermis, lie the layers of muscle and fatty tissue that support the overlying skin, giving it its firmness and determining its characteristic contour.

SKIN TYPES

Individual skin type is almost entirely a matter of genetic programming, with such characteristics as colouring, texture and susceptibility to allergy built into the DNA blueprint from the moment of conception. Although there are numbers of extremes and permutations, the principal skin types can be broken down as follows.

OILY SKIN, which often has a coarse grain with visible or open pores and a tendency to surface sheen, especially on the forehead, nose and chin, is more likely to develop acne, spots, blackheads, and other pore problems. Usually fairly tough and resilient, it is more resistant to the effects of ageing, including wrinkles, lines and creases, and is less likely to become dry and taut in extreme environmental conditions. It may be olive-toned and liable to tan without burning, or, at the other end of the spectrum, very sallow or ashy pale. Dandruff and excess facial hair may sometimes be problems which accompany excessive greasiness.

FAIR AND DRY SKIN, in contrast, appears relatively fine, even translucent, and may be more susceptible to allergies, dermatitis, tautness, itching and flaking, especially in very hot or cold weather. Apart from the face, the hands, shins and elbows, where skin is relatively thin and has no underlying sebaceous glands, are areas most prone to suffer from severe dryness. Fair, dry skin is usually thinner than its olive or oily counterpart, with a fine texture, almost invisible pores and little facial or body hair. It may have less underlying subcutaneous tissue and less active sweat and oil glands than oily or darker skin. Reduced skin secretions make dryness and premature wrinkles a particular problem.

Fair pink or peach-toned skin, especially when accompanied by blonde or red hair and blue, grey or green eyes, has relatively little melanin distribution, creating an increased risk of sunburn. Freckles, which may be visible at all times, or only materialize in sunlight, indicate that irregular 'clumps' of melanin are distributed throughout the epidermis. The thinner the skin, the more clearly the underlying veins and tiny capillaries may be visible, and broken red veins, as well as flushing or heightened skin colour, may be a particular problem, especially if aggravated by a faulty diet or environmental factors. In general, the fairer and dryer the skin, the greater the likelihood of allergies, irritation, eczema, sun damage and premature ageing.

ASIAN AND ORIENTAL SKINS probably suffer fewer endogenous problems than any other skin types. Resistant to degenerative changes, blemishes are the exception rather than the rule. Facial and body hair is sparse, the sweat and sebaceous glands tend to be relatively under-active, the texture is generally smooth, and pigmentation usually evenly and consistently distributed. The pigmentary anomalies that plague both white and black skin are, therefore, relatively rare.

BLACK SKINS, with their formidable pigmentary 'armour', have an inherent monopoly on youth, remaining unmarred by lines and wrinkles for longer than white skins largely because of a natural resistance to dryness, sun damage and the corrosive effects of the elements. However, when black skin does suffer injury, either through surgery, burns, lesions, or severe acne, it has an inbuilt tendency to heal imperfectly, forming unsightly hyperpigmented bunched keloid scars – the main reason why plastic surgeons and dermatologists are loath to perform surgical procedures, such as chemical peeling, dermabrasion or even electrolysis, on black skin. Pigmentary disorders such as vitiligo, whereby sometimes extensive areas of skin lose their normal colour, are also far more noticeable, and therefore distressing, to anyone with a black skin.

Probably the greatest hazard facing fashion-conscious black-skinned women, at present, is the large number of skin-bleaching creams and other agents on the market today. These can cause disastrous inflammatory side-effects, resulting in permanent damage, especially if used in a very hot, sunny climate.

CHANGING FORTUNES

Although the skin's basic profile and intrinsic temperament, how it reacts to internal biological change, as well as external influences, are largely laid down within each person's genetic blueprint, there are many extraneous factors which may either contribute positively to the condition of the skin or, conversely, can militate against both its healthy function and aesthetic appeal. Indeed, it is quite possible to be born with a relatively well-behaved, clear and radiant complexion, but eventually to end up, years later, with skin that has become so damaged through surface abuse, ill health, and faulty diet, that it bears little resemblance to its former flawless self. Perfect skin is not, as is sometimes believed, a legacy that necessarily endures for life. Likewise, judicious skin care, and in particular a regime that takes into account such internal factors as diet and stress, which dictate day-to-day skin function, can work wonders in reversing or at least ameliorating inherent chronic disorders. Thus, 'problem skin' is often far from being a *fait accompli*, a fate to which the sufferer has little option but to resign him- or herself. The relative health and beauty of skin is, therefore, something over which we do, in fact, have numerous opportunities to exert control.

The differences between healthy and unhealthy skin extend far beyond its surface. When caring for skin it is important to remember that, like physical wellbeing and the surrounding environment, skin is in a perpetual state of change, constantly adapting to the stimuli that arise from within and without. Therefore, whether your aim is to maintain and care for skin that is already in prime condition and doing you proud, or to try to improve on nature to the point of a complete overhaul, it is necessary first to recognize what makes skin tick. Which are the principal factors most likely to influence the day-to-day look and feel of your skin, for better or worse?

MOISTURE

When you consider that water accounts for roughly 55 per cent or more of a woman's body weight (65 per cent of a man's) and is the prime constituent of blood, lymph and tissue fluid, its importance in maintaining not just healthy skin but good health generally, becomes self-evident. Skin tissue is composed of 20 per cent water, therefore excessive dehydration or insufficient fluid intake is calculated to produce the most rapid and noticeable changes at all levels of the skin. When the stratum corneum (epidermis) lacks sufficient water to remain properly lubricated and flexible, dryness, cracking and roughness are the inevitable result.

The body loses, on average, 1.5 litres (2½ pints) water daily, much of this via the skin. Moisture is constantly evaporating imperceptibly from the skin's surface, through the process of transpiration, at the rate of about 500 ml (18 fl oz) per day, more in a very hot and dry environment. More noticeably, moisture is also being excreted through perspiration when, under extreme conditions, the sweat glands can pour out as much as 10 litres (18 pints) per day! Unless this loss is regularly replaced through adequate fluid intake, the skin will begin to look dry and 'pinched', developing surface lines and losing its elasticity.

Obviously, there are times when the body's fluid requirements become more urgent, for example immediately following vigorous physical exertion, during hot, dry weather, or when considerable amounts of fluid are lost through fever, vomiting and diarrhoea, which are often accompanied by excess sweating. There are other times when external or internal influences can create a short-term fluid 'crisis', resulting in temporary skin deterioration. For example, being subjected to atmospheric decompression during long-distance air travel makes tight, dry skin just one of the more obvious manifestations of jetlag, a condition exacerbated by drinking alcohol and large amounts of caffeine during the flight. Cigarette smoking, or even spending long periods in a confined smoke-laden environment, can rob the skin cells of vital nutrients because of the tendency for carbon monoxide temporarily to inactivate the blood's capacity to carry oxygen. Excessive alcohol consumption, apart from cluttering the system with toxic waste, rapidly depletes fluid levels and leads to dehydration as the body works overtime to metabolize alcohol and eliminate it from the system.

HORMONES

It is no coincidence that the skin can, at times, be so susceptible to periods of hormonal flux or imbalance. The action both of the male and female sex hormones – respectively known as androgens and oestrogen – can have a dramatic and far-reaching effect on the various skin systems. For evidence of this, one need only look at such problems chronologically.

ACNE
Development of acne, the severest hormone-linked disorder, coincides with the onset of puberty, the period of greatest hormonal upheaval. A massive outpouring, in both teenage boys and girls, of the principal male and female sex hormones not only initiates the development of primary and secondary sexual characteristics (body and facial hair, changes in voice, genitals and body contour), but may also lead to the scourge of adolescence – spotty infected skin. Very occasionally, an extreme imbalance of sex hormones can cause young women to develop excessive and unsightly facial and body hair.

Although the development and severity of acne seems to be largely determined by heredity and race (acne appears to be more common amongst white people and considerably less prevalent in racial groups such as the Japanese and those with black skins) and can be aggravated by environmental and physical factors, the underlying cause is increased sebaceous activity leading to blockage and inflammation of the hair follicles. Both these conditions seem to be triggered by increased hormonal activity. Doctors are agreed that most acne sufferers share one overriding characteristic, an abnormal sensitivity to the body's own production of androgens, principally the male sex hormone, testosterone, produced in very large quantities in males and in very small amounts in females. Interestingly, it is this same factor which is responsible for causing so-called 'male pattern baldness' in men of all ages.

By no means all individuals in their teens are condemned to suffer pimples, spots or oily skin problems, and the precise factors that predispose some people to suffer from acne until well into their twenties, even their thirties, while others go through their teens without a mark or blemish, remains rather a mystery. However, because of the various biological changes that can affect hormone production and thereby cause increased sebaceous activity and inflammatory reactions within the skin, it seems that stress, certain drugs and exposure to various chemicals may either trigger spots or aggravate existing acne. Excessive sebaceous activity is also one of the principal causes of seborrheic dermatitis, often accompanied by greasy hair and dandruff.

OESTROGEN-RELATED PROBLEMS
The hormonal changes that occur during pregnancy, the menopause or PMT (pre-menstrual tension), may all, in subtle and different ways, contribute to numerous transient skin problems, even in skin that is normally smooth, well behaved and problem free. Hormonal flux during the 14 days between ovulation and menstruation may create a tendency towards fluid retention, resulting in puffiness of the facial tissues and sensitivity or swelling of the legs, ankles, thighs and breasts. During pregnancy, the consistently high levels of oestrogen produced by the body may improve a woman's general skin condition, making her complexion appear noticeably smoother and more radiant. On the debit side, however, these hormonal changes can also cause parts of the skin to become more photosensitive, with the result that darkly pigmented patches, or 'chloasma', may develop on the forehead, upper lip and around the crests of the cheek bones during exposure to sunlight. In addition, the massive plummeting of hormone levels after childbirth may set the scene for any number of disorders, such as dryness, hair loss and flaking – problems that can also occur later in life during the menopause, when the ovaries cease their normal production of oestrogen.

Wrinkles, lines, excessive dryness, sagging and crêpiness, all due in part to diminished collagen synthesis, may all be associated with decreased oestrogen output, whether as a result of the menopause, having a complete hysterectomy (removal of womb and both ovaries), or amenorrhoea (the complete absence of regular periods) due to crash dieting, anorexia nervosa or very intensive vigorous physical exercise. Continuing research into causes and effects of one of the principal age-related ailments, osteoporosis (weak and brittle bones), common amongst post-menopausal women, is now beginning to point to a very close causal relationship between dwindling oestrogen levels and diminished collagen synthesis. It seems that loss of bone mass, accompanied by thinning and rapid ageing of skin, is a phenomenon researchers attribute in part to disintegration of collagen, the principal protein structure, as important a component of skin as it is of the matrix of joints and bones. Regular collagen synthesis, it seems, can only be maintained on a regular basis if oestrogen levels are sufficiently high, since the fibroblasts – the cells that manufacture collagen – have inbuilt oestrogen receptors that take up the hormone as part of their normal metabolic activity.

HORMONAL HICCUPS

Any imbalance in the function of the thyroid gland, responsible for activating the release of energy in the tissue from the combustion of glucose, may also contribute to skin problems. Dry, puffy skin and hair loss, accompanied by mental and physical lethargy and diminished appetite, are typical symptoms of reduced thyroid activity. Puffiness and swelling, associated with fluid retention, can be traced to any number of organic disorders, such as heart, liver or kidney disease, but a more frequent, less sinister, cause is so-called 'osmotic oedema' due to salt retention, usually as a result of sluggish kidney function or impaired circulation of blood through the kidneys leading to an accumulation of salt and excess water in the tissues.

The rate at which salt is passed in the urine is normally determined by the output of hormones secreted by all the adrenal glands. However, since the balance of the hormones is also determined by changing levels of female sex hormones during ovulation, menstruation and pregnancy, it is not surprising that fluid retention and puffiness should become more of a problem during these times. Fluid retention tends also to block the follicles, while changing hormone levels may increase the activity of the sebaceous glands, so that women with normally unblemished skin will suffer excess greasiness and acne just before or during menstruation.

CIRCULATION

Any subtle and gradual changes in skin texture and tone, such as the appearance of sallowness, clogged pores and pimples, are often an early indication that the body's main filtering systems, the lungs, kidneys or liver, are overloaded or blocked and are not functioning efficiently. The skin then becomes like an overflow. Similarly, if the circulatory system fails to deliver the regular fresh supplies of oxygen and nutrients necessary for efficient cell metabolism, then the consequences of malnourishment of the tissues is bound, sooner or later, to show up on the skin's surface. Any illness or medication that directly affects the kidneys, liver, blood circulation and lymph system, may ultimately be reflected in deterioration of the skin. However, such disruptive influences may not necessarily show up instantaneously, which explains why sudden 'mystery' skin disorders, apparently unlinked to ill-health, prove so very puzzling. It can take up to 21 days or longer for surface skin to renew itself completely, which accounts for the delay in externally visible signs of stress, pollution or organic malaise. Just as the effects of an illness or period of medication, crash dieting or unhealthy eating are often reflected in deterioration of the hair and nails weeks, even months, after the event, so the same time-lapse applies to skin.

EXERCISE

The perpetual repair, nourishment and building of new skin tissues cannot take place without a constant supply of oxygen-rich blood to the cells, the by-product of efficient circulation. Regular exercise, therefore, is a prerequisite for skin health and beauty since it not only boosts the blood supply to the skin, but also stimulates the flow of lymph, aiding the elimination of waste matter. There is little doubt that the skin of someone who takes plenty of vigorous aerobic exercise, much of it out of doors, tends to be clearer, firmer, more radiant and supple, due to improved muscle tone, than that of a person who is largely inactive. There is also growing evidence that physical exercise helps to maintain the youthful quality of the collagen and elastin structures within the dermis itself. According to studies carried out in Finland, comparing the skin of physically active athletes to that of ex-athletes who had stopped exercising, the connective tissue of those who exercised regularly was thicker and less subject to degenerative changes than of those who lived sedentary lives. When exercise stopped, however, this bonus was found to diminish along with fitness levels.

THE IMMUNE SYSTEM

Skin counts as the body's first line of defence against invasion by bacteria, virus or fungus. Could you see them, you would be able to count an average 100,000 microbes per square centimetre (½ inch) of skin, just one small sector of the resident 'home guard' all working in perpetual unison to attack and destroy potentially harmful foreign material. Apart from being an anti-bacterial screen, the hydrolipidic film, a blend of oils, salt, water and urea produced by the sweat glands, which covers the stratum corneum, also acts as a natural moisturizer, keeping the tissues soft and smooth. Slightly acidic in composition, this lipid barrier is susceptible to destruction by harsh alkaline chemicals. When the skin is particularly sensitive and the onslaught of chemicals very fierce or prolonged, resulting in significant damage, there is a very real danger that, being unprotected, the skin will become more vulnerable to infection, dryness, blisters, rashes and cracking, such as in severe cases of contact dermatitis and eczema.

Considering its role in combating infection, it is not surprising that the health and appearance of the skin are closely linked to the function of the body's immune system. The closeness of this relationship is only just beginning to emerge, albeit piecemeal, as a result of current research within the expanding and complex field of immunology. For example, one of the theories about the cause of atopic eczema, a skin disease which belongs to a group of inherited, so-called atopic, or allergic, conditions including asthma, hay fever and migraine, is that sufferers have an inbuilt kink or defect in their immune system which creates an inherited predisposition towards a wide variety of allergic reactions. The tendency for the body to manufacture excessive amounts of what are termed IgE antibodies in response to normally harmless substances such as household dust, animal fur, feathers, pollen, household chemicals and varieties of different foods, as well as during periods of emotional stress, is believed to be a predominant characteristic common to many eczema sufferers. Similarly, the immune system is also believed to be in some way implicated in chronic acne. Although shifting hormone levels, over-activity of the oil glands, and blocked follicles are known to be the main culprits, what still remains a mystery is why some people with very greasy skin and blackheads do not ever develop inflamed skin. Acne is a condition riddled with anomalies. One explanation is that the immune system of acne sufferers is pre-programmed to activate normally harmless bacteria that reside in the skin, causing them to break down excess oil into fatty acids, highly irritating substances that are largely to blame for the typical inflammatory nature of acne.

Eczema and acne are only two disorders seemingly associated with idiosyncrasies of the immune system. There are a variety of skin ailments, including thrush, boils, hives, warts and other sundry infections which tend to persist whenever immunity is weakened and the body cannot do a proper job in fighting off bacteria. Skin problems are, therefore, a common side effect of any drug treatment that affects the immune system, such as cortisone. Viral infections, including herpes, have been found to strike more readily when there is suppressed immune function, while one of the most classic, widespread symptoms of AIDS, a virus that heralds the total and fatal breakdown of the body's immune system, is an unsightly form of skin cancer called Karposi's sarcoma. The development of malignant melanoma, the most common and deadly form of skin cancer, normally associated with sun damage, is also believed to occur as a result of suppressed immune function. Numerous incurable mystery ailments like psoriasis and vitiligo (de-pigmented patches of skin on the face and body) are thought, on the other hand, to be auto-immune disorders, whereby the immune system fails to recognize certain of the body's own constituents and attacks that part of itself as if it were a foreign substance.

Although it doesn't give us the entire picture, impaired immunity does provide important missing links to the bewildering puzzle of many skin ailments, helping to explain why these first occur or are exacerbated at times of intense stress or emotional trauma. Although research is still in its infancy, there is growing conclusive evidence of the very powerful effect of the mind and emotions on body systems.

DAMAGE AND POLLUTION – THE EXTERNAL INFLUENCES

Well designed, tough and protective as it is, there are times when, by mere virtue of its accessibility, skin may be rendered perilously susceptible to environmental onslaught. Parts of the body, especially the face and hands, and any other areas that might be exposed, are particularly vulnerable to external influences. It is hardly surprising, therefore, that the ill effects of environmental extremes and chemical pollution should so affect the skin.

CITY SKIN – A MODERN HAZARD

Chemical pollution has become an all-pervasive hazard, particularly unavoidable for anyone living in big cities or highly built-up industrialized areas. Skin is a prime target for the noxious environmental substances that regularly assail us. Smog, petrol exhaust fumes, cigarette smoke, acid rain, ultraviolet radiation, man-made fabrics, modern household products, air conditioning, central heating, cosmetics, metals, and a myriad of different powerful chemicals now in routine domestic, office and industrial use, are just some of the everyday substances that can transform a normally benign environment into a potential danger zone for anyone with sensitive, allergy-prone skin.

The numbers of different synthetic chemicals known to cause contact dermatitis are legion. Particularly at risk are women working at home with harsh domestic products and those employed in specific professions, such as hairdressing, where the skin comes into continuous contact with corrosive or irritating substances. Luckily, however, most dermatitis sufferers, having once isolated and identified the substance or group of substances responsible for causing redness, dryness, itching or burning, are able either to avoid unnecessary contact with the offending product or can find ways to protect their skin and minimize the damage. Not surprisingly, the stress of not knowing the cause of a particular skin ailment, when added to the distress of having to endure painful unsightly rashes and eruptions, is probably also in part responsible for aggravating the condition.

The solution, however, is less simple when it comes to the less obvious 'invisible' allergens as well as the day-to-day environmental factors which we now take largely for granted as part and parcel of twentieth-century life. Though not harmful to skin in the majority of cases, there is increasing evidence to suggest that certain allergy-prone people, as well as those with inherently very temperamental skin, may fall victim to seemingly innocuous environmental factors. Take city grime, for example. The most obvious effect of urban living is the need for scrupulous skin cleansing to eliminate surface debris and grease, and to prevent sallowness, blackheads and clogged pores, which in turn can create a breeding ground for spots and pimples. Frequent bathing, showering, use of shampoos, soap, deodorants, anti-perspirants and skin lotions is, therefore, essential for maintaining good hygiene as well as ensuring fresh, clear-looking skin.

As well and good, but let's look at the possible rebound effects of over-zealous cleansing, a habit tempting for anyone who does not really feel fresh or comfortable unless they bathe, shower or scrub thoroughly perhaps two or three times daily. The irritant drying effects of many soaps, shampoos and skin tonics, as well as the abrasive effects men may experience through daily shaving and the problems associated with hard water, mean that anyone with characteristically dry skin runs the risk of dehydrating the surface tissues even further. In turn, this may cause itching, flaking, redness and heightened sensitivity to cold winds, sunlight and central heating, while making the skin appear taut, lined and raw. Conversely, scrubbing very oily, acne-prone skin can stimulate the oil glands to become more active, thus aggravating related skin disorders. Excessive use of deodorants and anti-perspirants, usually composed of strong chemical compounds, including aluminium salts, may cause itching, irritation or a more severe reaction.

THE BIG OUTDOORS

In contrast to dirt, however, the elements, at their most extreme, can exert very definite and noticeable changes within skin that is constantly exposed. Greasy, spotty skin may react adversely to hot, humid weather, becoming more oily and liable to outbreaks of cysts, boils or pimples if the follicles become blocked or inflamed. An additional hazard is that yeast and other fungal infections flourish under very warm, moist conditions, disturbing the normally balanced ecology of the skin, making it liable to attract and harbour any variety of unwelcome bacteria. This can be a particular problem if the immune system is suppressed for some reason.

Dryness, flaking and redness, chapped or cracked lips and splitting of the cuticles around the nails, are directly attributable to icy cold temperatures, keen winds and very dry, hot and sunny atmospheres, all of which relentlessly rob the uppermost tissues of vital stores of moisture unless properly protected with moisturizing creams. In fact, indoors or out, dry environments are a killer as far as the skin's surface is concerned. Particularly lethal are the sudden and extreme changes in temperature which may occur between indoor and outdoor environments, as is common, for instance, in winter when going from a very overheated shop or office into the freezing outdoors or, in summer, when temperatures of 25–35°C (80–90°F) are offset by air conditioning set at seemingly near-Arctic levels.

Once again, skin which is by nature delicate and intrinsically dry, stands the greatest chance of becoming taut, lined and ultrasensitive to such onslaughts of climatic highs and lows. By irritating the mucous membranes and the epithelial tissues lining the eyes, mouth and nose, dry air and climatic extremes can also cause itching and swelling of the facial tissues, sometimes accompanied by sinus inflammation or allergic rhinitis. Other factors, such as an unbalanced diet, cigarette smoking, drinking alcohol, illness and medication (especially the use of corticosteroid skin ointment) can contribute further to the effects of environmental dehydration. Although little can be done to mitigate the effects of dry, outdoor atmospheres, hot or cold, the humidity levels indoors should not, ideally, fall far short of 55–60 per cent to maintain the health and comfort of the skin and mucous membranes. Apart from using protective skin creams, drinking plenty of water, fruit juice or herbal tea and avoiding very salty or spicy food and drink can also help to replenish body fluids that are lost in extremely dry conditions.

OXIDATION AND CROSS-LINKING

Although tremendous controversy surrounds the issue of how and why we age, some researchers believe that exposure to high levels of pollution, whether from outside or inside the body, can accelerate the ageing process leading to premature degenerative changes in the skin. When inhaled, substances such as lead, cadmium, mercury, carbon monoxide and other noxious chemicals, including ozone, a prime constituent of urban smog, are broken down to form destructive chemicals known as 'free-radicals' believed to cause oxidation damage to the tissues and to hasten cellular ageing. These chemical pollutants are believed to be a principal contributory factor in a degenerative process called 'cross-linking' which is also the process that causes iron to go rusty, paper to turn yellow, celluloid to fade, rubber to become perished – and ultimately the whole of the human body to become less efficient and lose its youthful appearance. Thus, wrinkles, lines, creases, loss of firmness and suppleness, brown age spots, dehydration and sagging, represent the net effect of the inexorable process of oxidation and cross-linking of the skin's collagen and elastin fibres. Oxidation, however, is a normal effect of oxygen consumption and therefore of everyday living, inseparable from each and every one of the vital biological processes that keep us alive. It is therefore virtually impossible to prevent the insidious takeover of cells and tissues by chemical invaders, except by living in a relatively unpolluted environment and avoiding such obvious internal pollutants as alcohol, cigarette smoke, drugs and processed 'junk' foods. Some clinical ecologists believe the ill effects of these chemicals can be greatly offset by stepping up the intake of specific nutrients like beta carotene, vitamins A, C, E and the trace element selenium which, because they contain anti-oxidant properties, may protect the tissues from damage.

SICK OFFICE SKIN

Not surprisingly, those prone to allergies and chronic skin problems, such as eczema or psoriasis, stand to fear the most from atmospheric pollution at its most concentrated. Many sufferers discover their condition becomes worse during exposure to very polluted smog- or smoke-laden atmospheres, while redness, burning and itching are frequent even amongst those with no inherent disorder. Office workers with hyper-sensitive skin are particularly liable to become victims of the so-called 'sick office' syndrome. Carbonless copying paper, photocopying materials, correcting and cleaning fluids, are just some of the many substances commonly used nowadays in offices that have been implicated as the cause of skin rashes. Amongst the many different reported ill effects suffered by users of VDUs, such as tiredness, headaches and eye problems, are skin dryness, scaliness, spots, sensitivity and redness, including the so-called 'three o'clock flush', which is a distinctive reddening of the face late in the afternoon, presumably due to having spent the greater part of the day face-to-face with a word processor or computer. The symptoms are believed to be due to the electrostatic field set up by the VDU, causing charged particles and contaminants to settle on the face. When ventilation is inadequate, and humidity levels in the office are, as is common, already very low and the levels of static correspondingly high, there is a good chance the skin will become more readily sensitized. Other predisposing factors with a tendency to sensitize the skin, are highly spiced foods, alcohol and excessive caffeine, all of which should be avoided by anyone suffering from any form of office-related skin problems.

SUNLIGHT

Though some amount of sunshine is vital for proper synthesis of Vitamin D, and thus the formation of healthy bone and tissues, in excess ultraviolet light represents potentially the single greatest environmental enemy of human skin. What is more, the nature of the damage wrought to skin by excessive strong sunlight, is such that it is well nigh irreversible, nor can the destructive influence of ultraviolet light be greatly mitigated by such internal factors as diet, because the sun's rays do not merely affect surface tissues but act as a catalyst deep down within the dermal layers, transforming the function and structure of living tissue.

On a visible level, the causal relationship between strong sunlight and skin damage is self evident, particularly amongst those with fair, so-called Celtic skins, endowed with very small stores of melanin necessary to produce a protective sun-tan. Burning, swelling, blistering and peeling are the most obvious and instantaneous effects of too much exposure to the sun. The links between repeated sunburn and the tough, coarse, leathery and mottled skins of men and women who have spent their youth and middle years devoted to indiscriminate sun worship, have long been proven without any shadow of a doubt. In-depth analysis of the skin of people living in very hot, sunny countries, proves conclusively that collagen and elastin fibres cross-link and break down prematurely and more dramatically while the skin becomes steadily more susceptible to broken red veins, lines and brown age spots than is normal amongst those who live in less sunny climes and assiduously protect their skin from sunlight.

Dermatologists are unequivocal in their condemnation of too much sunlight as the single most potent cause of premature skin ageing. If those with fair dry skin suffer the worst, those with greasy skin don't necessarily fare so well either. Although acne and other blemishes may clear up temporarily after initial exposure to sunlight, long periods spent in very intense heat and strong sun can, paradoxically, aggravate spots and pimples by stimulating the oil glands while clogging up the follicles with dry, hardened particles of skin. Allergic skin conditions, in particular acne rosacea, inevitably flare up in strong sunlight and the recurrence of cold sores around the mouth often coincides with periods of very hot sunny weather.

In addition to these obvious hazards, there are numerous variables that can determine the way skin reacts to the sun. Medication is one typical example. The contraceptive pill, tranquillizers, diuretics, certain antibiotics and anti-fungal pills are all known to cause photosensitivity in certain people, resulting in rashes, burns or brown blotches on the face or body. Some artificial sweeteners, such as saccharine, and halogenated salicylamides, an ingredient used in deodorant soaps, may also cause an adverse reaction. The juice of certain fruits and vegetables, especially those high in psoralens – a known photosensitizing agent – including limes, figs, celery, parsley and parsnips, especially if eaten in excess prior to sunbathing, may cause burning or blotchiness, while applying certain cosmetics and perfumes, especially those containing oil of bergamot, a potent sensitizer, may interact badly with ultraviolet light, whether the source is natural sunlight or a sunbed.

SKIN CANCER

More sinister by far, however, than the ageing aspect, is the latest evidence of the relationship between sunlight and skin cancer. Virtually endemic amongst fair-skinned men and women living an active outdoor life in countries such as New Zealand, Australia and South Africa, the incidence of skin cancer and pre-cancerous growths (solar keratoses) per capita is doubled every 200 miles nearer the Equator. Those of us who live in relatively temperate, unsunny countries in the Northern hemisphere, may therefore feel tempted to adopt an attitude of complacency. Yet we do so at our peril.

Recent research suggests that the incidence in Britain of the deadliest form of skin cancer, malignant melanoma, which now represents 2 per cent of all cancers, and 1 per cent of all cancer deaths, has more than doubled in the last 10 years, a trend dermatologists believe coincides with an increase in holidays taken abroad in the Mediterranean and other hot, sunny countries when the skin is exposed each year to a short, sharp but intensive blast of strong sunlight. Sadly, it seems that skin damage caused through sunburn and prolonged exposure to the sun need only take place a few times before certain degenerative changes begin to occur within the tissues and, more specifically and seriously, within the DNA of individual skin cells. It is the power of ultraviolet light to initiate subtle mutations within the cells, thus altering their capacity to repair themselves and reproduce in a correct, healthy fashion, which accounts for the most serious potential danger of sunlight. Apart from causing degenerative changes like blemishes, keratoses and benign growths, skin cells that are inherently defective and reproduce incorrectly almost certainly constitute the root cause of skin cancer. In addition, there is growing evidence to suggest that prolonged exposure to ultraviolet light also lowers the body's immune defence system, another possible contributory factor in the development of cancer.

Ultraviolet light consists principally of two wavebands, shortwave UVB rays which burn the skin, damaging the uppermost tissues, and longwave UVA rays responsible for tanning and which, until recently, were regarded as relatively weak and harmless. The ideal safe strategy for sun lovers might therefore seem simple – get tanned, but don't get burned. Today, sun worshippers need to think again. Sunburn is not necessarily, as it now turns out, always the sole precursor to eventual longterm degenerative damage. Sunlight wreaks much of its damage in a slow, stealthy manner. The effects, at first virtually imperceptible, tend to be cumulative. What is more, those ultraviolet rays that penetrate into the dermis, stimulating melanin production, are those hitherto allegedly 'safe' longwave UVA rays which also have the power to dig deepest into the living heart of the cell – the DNA. Those people who normally tan easily without discomfort or burning, may consequently be just as liable to tissue changes on a deep level, resulting in premature ageing and possibly more serious disorders, even cancer.

There is no doubt, therefore, that in order to avoid all forms of skin degeneration you should ideally try to stay out of strong sunlight altogether or else protect the skin with a good quality sunscreen or sunblock which effectively filters out both UVB and UVA rays. Another important point to remember is that surfaces such as concrete, snow, white walls, water, even pale sand, can reflect the sun's rays, increasing their intensity and ability to harm the skin.

HOLES IN THE OZONE LAYER

The facts, therefore, speak for themselves. To retain a youthful, healthy skin avoid undue exposure to sunlight. So far so good. But do we – or will we in the coming years – always have the choice? In the light of all the current findings about the effects of sunlight, one emerging environmental trend is particularly alarming – the gradual depletion of the earth's protective ozone layer which screens out the strongest and most damaging rays emitted by the sun. It has been estimated that if there is a continuing decline in the ozone layer, due largely to the release of chlorofluorocarbon (CFC) gases which puncture 'holes' in the earth's atmosphere, the risk of developing skin cancer could rise by one-third over the next 40 years, both by affecting the body's immune system and by damaging skin tissue. Covering up as much as possible is one answer; using effective sun screening agents all the year round, not just during the summer, is clearly another, for anyone wishing to minimize the possible ill effects of ultraviolet radiation. A third tactic is obviously to ensure that the immune system does not become weakened or defective through undue stress, taking drugs, and developing nutritional deficiencies as a result of eating an unbalanced diet.

SUN 'STARVATION' – EFFECTS OF ULTRAVIOLET DEPRIVATION

With today's mounting alarm over excessive ultraviolet radiation, it is all too easy to overlook what happens when, as in a minority of cases, skin is not exposed sufficiently to sunlight, the prime source of Vitamin D and essential for the growth of strong, healthy bones, teeth, muscle and other tissue. Although it is rare nowadays for children and adults not to receive adequate ultraviolet light stimulus, theoretically anyone who gets up in the morning while it is still dark, spends all day indoors in a dim artificially lit environment, goes home when it is dark or goes to bed early at night, runs the risk of Vitamin D deficiency linked to insufficient sunlight. Wearing clothes that cover up most of the body, throughout the entire year, can further militate against the absorption of ultraviolet light. There is evidence, also, that adults and children with black skin cannot synthesize Vitamin D as readily as those with white skin, because increased levels of pigmentation act as a natural sun screen, cutting down the rate at which the skin converts ultraviolet light to Vitamin D. Black, Asian or Oriental children and adults living in countries within the northern hemisphere, particularly in cities that are smog-laden and very built up, where the winters are long and relatively unsunny, and the summers often overcast, stand the greatest risk of developing rickets and osteomalacia, the principal symptoms of Vitamin D deficiency.

White skin is at an advantage because it allows between 53 and 72 per cent of ultraviolet light to pass far enough into the dermis to trigger Vitamin D synthesis. Black skins, however, allow only between 3 and 36 per cent to pass through to this layer, which means a large percentage of Vitamin D must come instead from dietary sources such as dairy produce and fish. An additional danger with certain ethnic groups is the custom of women and children to cover up virtually the entire body, and sometimes even the face, throughout the year, while spending much time indoors, two factors which can drastically limit the amount of sunshine that gets to the body. Softening of the bones is often a problem, therefore, amongst Muslim women in India and Pakistan, where veils are still worn and both calcium and Vitamin D are notably absent from the diet. Eskimos, who have a relatively dark complexion and live most of their lives covered in thick, warm clothing, obtain most of their Vitamin D requirements from a diet incorporating large quantities of oily fish.

INTERNAL INFLUENCES – PSYCHOLOGY AND MOOD

As we have seen, the condition of the skin is closely allied to bodily health and wellbeing. Emotions and moods of all sorts can affect the skin, which acts almost as a mirror, reflecting the inner state.

STRESS

Since there is hardly an organ or function which is not in some way affected by stress, it is little wonder that the skin so often bears the imprint of inner conflict or emotional shock, as well as prolonged tiredness, tension and trauma.

From conception onwards, the skin and nervous system are closely inter-related. During the first stage of embryonic development, the cells which later help to form, the skin, hair and nails, as well as the pituitary and adrenal glands – the key sites of nervous activity – all make up the ectoderm which in effect constitutes the embryo during its first eight weeks of development. From then on, until birth, the rate and stages of development of the skin and spinal cord remain in close synchrony. The appendages of skin – hair and nails – made up of the same keratinous protein substance as the epidermis, often provide the earliest visible signs of the extent to which physical appearance mirrors psychological turmoil. Falling hair, greasiness, dryness, flaking or itching of the scalp, or splitting, weak or brittle nails are typical indicators that the body is under stress.

The effects of stress on skin can be either immediate, as in the case of eczema or hives, or delayed, as for example with viral infections, depending on the source and nature of the stress to which a person is subjected. Nervous tension, by activating the body's automatic fight or flight response, can cause excessive sweating and increased muscle tension, which in turn narrows the underlying blood vessels, reducing the flow of blood to the tissues, and increases the activity of the oil glands. All of these reflex actions, directly controlled by the so-called 'sympathetic' branch of the body's automatic nervous system, have fairly rapid and sometimes visible effects on the skin's outward appearance. Extreme pallor, sometimes interspersed with flushing, sweating or greasiness, are the main outward indicators of bodily arousal. But it is beneath the skin's surface that the major adaptive forces come into play. In response to messages of fear, anger, aggression, anxiety, nervousness or pain, registered by the brain, the hypothalamus gland, in close collaboration with its number two, the pituitary gland, sends prompt instructions to the adrenal glands to pump massive supplies of stress hormones, including adrenalin, noradrenalin and cortisol into the bloodstream. The instant effect of these chemicals is to increase the heartbeat, to raise blood pressure and oxygen consumption, and to close down all the digestive processes by shunting blood away from the stomach and towards the muscles for extra strength. Glycogen stored in the liver is released as glucose sugar to provide adequate sources of instant energy. The body's stores of protein and fat are similarly broken down and discharged into the system while the output of the body's own anti-inflammatory chemicals rises, simultaneously suppressing the function of the immune system. This all-out 'red alert' is the same whether the source of stress is relatively welcome, for instance when sexually attracted to someone, or nerve-racking as when faced with a competition or exam, or indeed, profoundly distressing, as is the case during conflict at home or work, a serious illness, bereavement or accident.

The fight or flight response per se is perfectly normal and healthy – indeed a necessary factor of survival – provided it doesn't continue uninterruptedly for very long periods. However, so diverse and numerous are the potential sources of stress in the modern world, that it is today regarded as a major contributory factor in the development of a wide spectrum of chronic degenerative and life-threatening illnesses, including heart disease, hypertension, cancer, ulcers, and other gastric ailments. Its effects on different organs and functions of the body mean that prolonged or very severe stress can be largely to blame for causing or aggravating numerous chronic disorders, such as migraine, backache, asthma, phobias, depression, menstrual and premenstrual disorders, sexual dysfunctions and, of course, skin problems. Chronic complaints like acne, herpes, eczema and psoriasis very often first occur, or else are exacerbated, during periods of extreme stress or emotional trauma. Studies conducted in the USA indicate that a large percentage of teenage acne sufferers experience a deterioration in the skin just prior to and during school exams. One of the theories is that stress raises levels of the male sex hormone, testosterone, which also exists in very small amounts in women, and which in certain individuals causes the follicles and oil ducts to become inflamed. Less common mystery ailments, like vitiligo (de-pigmentation), also sometimes appear to be triggered during a time of emotional upheaval.

The exact mechanism by which stress alters the function and structure of skin remains very much a dermatological imponderable. What seems likely, however, is that by exacerbating inflammatory processes, suppressing the immune system, creating nutritional deficiencies, in particular lowering the amounts of B complex vitamins, vitamin C and zinc in the body, and also altering the normal levels of certain hormones, the skin may inevitably suffer, if only in an indirect, roundabout way.

Even though we do not know, as yet, what exact biochemical ups and downs may jeopardize the skin's condition, there are other easily indentifiable factors that go hand in hand with a stressful lifestyle, and which can all too easily contribute to skin problems: cigarette smoking; drinking too much alcohol, strong coffee or tea; insufficient sleep, rest or exercise; taking hard drugs or tranquillizers; becoming dependent on 'comfort foods' such as sweets, chocolates and biscuits; eating an unbalanced diet high in fats, sugar and processed foods; crash dieting or else developing eating disorders, such as anorexia or bulimia nervosa. These are all habits associated with stress, and calculated to wreak some form of damage to the skin.

PSYCHE AND SKIN – THE HIDDEN LINK

Mood, whether on a noticeable conscious level or representing conflicts hidden away in the deepest recesses of the subconscious, may also, subtly yet significantly, cause shifts in physical wellbeing, including the health of the skin. If happiness and inner calm or wellbeing are often reflected in a radiant complexion, then depression and anxiety just as predictably are associated with the skin that looks pallid and lacklustre. The numbers of psoriasis and eczema sufferers who have obtained considerable improvement, even a complete cure, as a result of resolving emotional conflicts, reducing the tension in their lives, and becoming mentally more optimistic, positive and cheerful, indicate that the theory of a link between the psyche and the skin is not merely idle conjecture.

Some psychotherapists even claim that trauma or severe shock dating back to childhood and perhaps long forgotten or suppressed, may surface, quite literally, in the form of periodic or persistent skin eruptions, especially when the sufferer is under extra emotional strain. Just as asthma, digestive upsets or phobias often have their origins in early childhood experience, recurring later on in life at times of stress, so skin may also be the target organ that bears the brunt of inner, unresolved turmoil, or negative self-defeating emotions, such as guilt, fear and anger, which cannot be fully expressed or exorcised. Patients suffering from chronic skin disorders, who obtain professional help in the form of counselling, hypnotherapy, or other forms of psychotherapy, to help them handle stress more effectively and overcome many of their emotional problems, often report that their condition coincidentally also improves, even disappearing for long periods altogether as they follow a more balanced and harmonious life style.

THE INSIDE INFORMATION – POLLUTION, DRUGS AND DIET

For better or for worse, the basic condition of skin is ultimately largely dependent on what goes on inside the body and on the substances that filter through into the very deepest layers of the skin. Surface skin is, after all, merely the outer casing, the finished product resulting from numerous complex and lengthy biochemical changes and finely synchronized processes. Just as truly healthy problem-free skin is largely a by-product of all-round bodily and emotional health, so the most disruptive influences are those which occur not from without but from within, upsetting hormone production, weakening immune function and sometimes leading to dehydration, inflammation, infection and toxic build-up.

CIGARETTES AND ALCOHOL

Cigarette smoking and heavy alcohol consumption are, without doubt, the two most potent forms of self-induced internal pollution. Both alcohol and tobacco permeate the tissues with a wide range of noxious pollutants, most of them powerful oxidizing agents, and therefore a potent force in the process of cross-linking and skin ageing. Quite apart from their harmful action on skin tissue, the potentially devastating effects of both substances on vital organic functions have been conclusively proven.

SMOKING

Lung cancer, emphysema and heart disease apart, smoking is also a prime enemy of the skin's natural beauty. On a purely mechanical level, the habit of smoking is likely to cause premature facial ageing as a result of the repeated frowning and grimacing involved in puffing, sucking, exhaling, inhaling, and lighting up cigarettes. These facial habits are largely responsible for causing those furrows around the lips, frown lines and crows' feet that are common in so many heavy smokers, especially those with a dry delicate skin.

The ageing process also goes on deeper within the dermis itself. Cigarette smoke produces numerous potent toxic substances including arsenic, tar, carbon monoxide, acetaldehyde and benzopyrene, which apart from hastening the oxidation of the tissues, have also been found to use up the body's supply of vitamin C, a vital substance in the repair and synthesis of healthy collagen. Smokers have been found to have lower than normal levels of vitamin C in their blood, a deficiency which may require several extra hundred milligrams of vitamin C per day to correct. Smoking is also responsible for depleting the B complex group of vitamins. Another reason why the skin of smokers often appears coarse and relatively dry is because the noxious gases also constrict the tiny blood vessels of the skin and reduce the oxygen-carrying capacity of the blood, thereby starving the tissues of vital nutrients.

ALCOHOL

In contrast to smoking, alcohol, if taken in moderation, say one or two glasses of wine a day, is believed to have certain beneficial effects on the body, improving digestion, aiding relaxation, dilating the blood vessels and so improving the circulation of blood to the tissues and protecting the heart. Taken in small quantities, alcohol also appears to raise the levels of high-density lipoproteins (HDL) in the blood, which help to counteract the potential ill effects of blood cholesterol. However, the hazards of drinking too much alcohol need little elaboration. Impaired liver function, leading to cirrhosis, shrinkage of the brain cells, diminished memory and co-ordination, depression and obesity are just some of the most serious effects of excess alcohol intake. Moreover, the virtually total systematic destruction of vitamins, minerals, trace elements, amino acids and other nutrients by alcohol is as mercilessly undiscriminating as it is unceasing. To drink too much is virtually to guarantee malnourishment of one degree or another, the effects of which invariably show up on the skin's surface. Worth remembering too, is the particular vulnerability of women to the effects of alcohol, mainly because of their inability to metabolize it as rapidly or efficiently as men, a disparity due mainly to reduced body size and a greater proportion of fatty tissue. Deficiencies of vitamins B_1, B_2, B_3, B_6, B_{12} and C, folic acid, calcium, magnesium and zinc are particularly marked amongst people who drink heavily, resulting in dehydration and wrinkling and impairment of the ability of skin tissue to heal properly after injury.

In the process of metabolizing alcohol and eliminating its toxic by-products from the system, the body needs to use up large extra quantities of fluid with the result that the tissues rapidly become dehydrated. Only by drinking six to eight glasses of water, or preferably vitamin C-rich fruit juice, after a bout of heavy alcohol consumption is it possible to prevent the skin from acquiring that coarse, grainy, dry and lined appearance so typical of the 'morning after the night before'.

Alcohol also interferes with the body's ability to metabolize a substance called cis-linoleic acid, one of the group of essential fatty acids necessary for the maintenance of healthy nerve, brain and skin tissue. In excess, it can have particularly detrimental effects on skin which is relatively thin and prone to redness, allergic reactions, broken red 'spider' veins or acne rosacea, a condition characterized by acute perpetual redness, lumps, bumps and broken capillaries. Sufferers are notoriously susceptible to the sensitizing effects of sunlight, extremes of hot and cold air, very spicy food, and alcohol, all of which cause the already congested and weakened blood vessels of the face to dilate and even rupture even further, and the skin's sensitive surface to become irritated and inflamed. By lowering the body's immune system, heavy drinking may also increase susceptibility to infections, including herpes, thrush, cysts and boils.

TEA AND COFFEE

Although there is little danger that drinking large amounts of coffee or tea will directly harm the skin, both beverages are high in so-called xanthines, stimulants such as caffeine, which cause nervous tension, irritability, sleeplessness and inability to relax. Drinking vast quantities of very strong coffee, in particular, often accompanies other symptoms of stressful living, such as smoking, eating an unbalanced diet and drinking too much alcohol.

By cranking up the body's production of stress hormones even further, too much caffeine may contribute to the whole vicious spiral of stress, itself sometimes being responsible for triggering stress-linked disorders like nervous eczema. Tea and coffee also have a strong diuretic action so there is a risk that bodily dehydration may be reflected on the skin's surface. Drinking tea or coffee at mealtimes can also reduce the amount of iron absorbed from vegetables to about one-third, obviously a problem for anyone liable to iron-deficiency anaemia, and can also inhibit zinc absorption, a factor sometimes associated with slow tissue healing. The many different chemicals present in tea and coffee may act as an irritant in some very sensitive, allergy-prone individuals, aggravating existing conditions, including psoriasis. As the main action of any stimulant, such as caffeine or alcohol, is to widen the blood vessels and increase circulation, strong tea or coffee should be avoided by anyone suffering from acne rosacea, severe flushing or chronic facial redness caused by overdilated, weak or ruptured capillary walls. As they have a destructive effect on the capillaries, very hot beverages of any type are best avoided by individuals with a skin problem linked to defective blood vessels.

MEDICATION

There are numerous drugs in existence, designed to treat diverse illnesses and conditions, which may significantly alter body chemistry, creating a heightened risk of skin disorders. By depleting the body's important nutrients, such as the B complex vitamins, vitamin C and zinc, there are some drugs which appear to pose more of a direct threat to the skin. Most ironic of all, however, is the fact that the very drugs commonly prescribed nowadays to treat certain skin disorders may sometimes cause untold longterm damage to the overall condition of the skin.

ANTIBIOTICS
Antibiotics are a mixed blessing as far as the skin goes. Frequently prescribed in low doses, but over prolonged periods, to treat acne, there is little doubt as to their effectiveness in reducing the underlying inflammation and so controlling cysts, boils and pustules. But at what cost? Recognized side-effects during therapy include the risk of photosensitivity, vaginal thrush and the possibility of a 'rebound' outbreak of acne, often in a more virulent form, once therapy has ended. In the end, antibiotics seem to work mainly by suppressing the symptoms, rather than effecting a complete cure or correcting the biochemical processes that cause inflammation. Doctors, however, maintain that provided the dosage is kept to a minimum and treatment carefully monitored, antibiotic therapy may result in longterm improvement without side-effects. Since even a very short course of antibiotics usually causes deficiencies of the B complex vitamins and alters the ecological balance of intestinal flora which protect against infection, the diet should be particularly high in wholefoods and fresh vegetables to guard against depression, fatigue, skin dryness and other symptoms of B

complex deficiency. Eating regular daily amounts of live yogurt helps to prevent antibiotics from destroying too many of the beneficial, protective bacteria in the gut, responsible for fighting off fungal infections.

Another much touted acne cure – 13-cis retinoic acid (also known as isotretinoin), a powerful synthetic vitamin A derivative, is also proving highly effective in controlling acne because of its ability to inhibit sebaceous secretions and reduce inflammation, but, again, the drug is not without its unwelcome side-effects. As might be expected with a substance that effectively limits the activity of the oil glands, the side-effects include dryness, itching of all the membranes – eyes, mouth and nasal passages – chafing of the lips, nosebleeds, muscle and joint ache. Unsuitable for pregnant women, the drug also elevates the level of blood fats, including cholesterol, which means that treatment must be carefully medically monitored.

THE CONTRACEPTIVE PILL

Prescription of the contraceptive pill to combat acne is no longer regarded as a viable alternative to antibiotic or retinoic acid therapy. For one thing, levels of oestrogen must be relatively high in order to have any effect on testosterone, the male sex hormone produced in small but significant amounts in women. In the light of recent evidence linking high-oestrogen contraceptives to certain forms of cancer, such treatment clearly poses unacceptably high health risks. Another reason why the contraceptive pill is no longer a feasible proposition as an anti-acne therapy, is that today's improved low-risk contraceptive pills contain relatively small amounts of oestrogen coupled with relatively large amounts of progestogen, a synthetic version of the female sex hormone progesterone, which does not successfully inhibit testosterone. On the contrary, it may, because of its relative affinity with the male sex hormone, aggravate inflammatory processes within the tissues. This may explain why taking the progestogen-only 'mini' pill can cause outbreaks of spots in some women.

Acne apart, taking the contraceptive pill can cause some women to develop chloasma, dark muddy-brown patches on the face, neck or chest that generally appear as a result of exposure to strong sunlight. Usually concentrated around the eye sockets, across the forehead and upper lip, chloasma, also known as the 'mask of pregnancy', is thought to be the direct result of heightened oestrogen and progesterone levels which, in turn, stimulate increased yet irregular melanin synthesis. Once the marks have developed, whether as a result of being pregnant or from taking the contraceptive pill, getting rid of them is fiendishly difficult, if not impossible. Using a complete sunblock all the time is one way of preventing them from spreading or becoming darker. Regular use of a hydroquinone-based skin bleaching cream may help to fade the patches, but hydroquinone itself may sensitize the skin, especially in very cold weather, causing redness and irritation.

CORTICOSTEROIDS – THE GREAT DESTROYERS

As far as the skin is concerned, potentially the most destructive of all forms of medication, whether taken internally or applied externally, are corticosteroid drugs, synthetic derivatives of hydrocortisone. These are often prescribed in very large quantities on an ongoing basis to control chronic inflammatory illnesses such as arthritis. The principal, and most serious, side-effect is the suppressive action of the drug on the adrenal glands, resulting in lowered immune function. Apart from leading to numerous possible infections and health complications, the effect of this on skin is often to cause excess facial hair, as well as any number of skin infections, including boils, fungal rashes, thrush or herpes. Diminished collagen synthesis, coupled with destruction of the delicate capillary walls in turn leads to increased bruising, broken 'spider' veins, flushing and delayed wound healing. Corticosteroids also alter the salt/potassium balance of the body, causing fluid retention and puffiness of the tissues due to excess salt and potassium deficiency.

Far more potentially damaging to the health and aesthetic appeal of the skin, however, are the topical corticosteroid ointments which are widely used to treat inflammatory skin diseases, principally eczema, dermatitis, psoriasis and even acne. Used over a prolonged period in high concentrations, their principal destructive action is to thin and eventually atrophy the skin's surface, weakening and rupturing the underlying collagen and elastin fibres causing wrinkling, sagging, diminished elasticity and stretch marks, as well as an expanding network of broken, ruptured red veins and translucent patches which become hypersensitive and allegy-prone. Sadly, the reason why these ointments are so popular amongst both doctors and patients, and thus widely over-prescribed, is precisely because of their initial success in eliminating inflammation. This apparent 'success' is, however, regrettably shortlived. Patients who have undergone longterm corticosteroid ointment therapy for eczema or psoriasis, especially where the ointment is applied continuously to the same areas of the face or body, may eventually discover, too late, that their skin has become 'hooked' on the product and, when treatment ceases, suffer a massive flaring up, in effect a rebound response, of the original condition. Many sufferers go on to develop allergic reactions to any number of stimuli, including sunlight, extremes of heat or cold, hot spicy food and drink, whereby the skin, now irredeemably sensitized, fragile and thin and lacking its normal protective, antibacterial lipid barrier, tends to burn, swell up or break out in spots, lumps and bumps – a condition sometimes known as iatrogenic (ie drug-induced) rosacea. If applied in excess, corticosteroid ointments can also permeate the epidermis, becoming absorbed by the body to the point where the active ingredient will have similar suppressive effects on the adrenal glands and immune system as when the drug is taken internally. Anyone embarking on a course of corticosteroid therapy should therefore take care to eat a well-balanced diet high in all the nutrients essential to proper immune function, while avoiding strong stimulants such as alcohol, spices, tea or coffee which may further irritate the skin.

NUTRITION: THE INSIDE STORY

Healthy, good-looking skin is inevitably created and maintained from within. Balanced nutrition is therefore the starting point for any in-depth skincare regime. Just as the quality of the food we eat is a major contributory factor towards our physical and psychological wellbeing, so, directly or indirectly, the right or wrong diet can subtly influence numerous aspects of the skin's structure and functions.

One obvious, extreme example of a direct association between diet and skin can be seen in the rashes and other allergic reactions which may flare up in response to eating individual or groups of 'trigger foods'. Another is the way in which skin becomes the eventual target of certain nutritional deficiencies or excesses, especially where these involve key nutrients (ie vitamin C, vitamin A or zinc) integral to the formation of healthy tissue.

An unbalanced diet is also likely to affect the skin in a more circuitous, altogether insidious manner, not always easy to recognize, by affecting those organs and processes that share certain biochemical mechanisms in common with the skin, or are directly implicated in the synthesis of skin cells. Given the structural complexity of the skin, and its close relationship with other organs as well as the diversity of its functions, sooner or later any nutritional imbalance, shortage or overload is bound to register on the surface or beneath, within the dermal tissues. Proper skincare is therefore synonymous with balanced nutrition which, by definition, should include as wide a variety of fresh, unprocessed foods as possible to provide all the vitamins, minerals, trace elements, protein, carbohydrate, fibre and fat necessary for good health. No single food or group of foods can adequately supply the body's entire needs.

All nutrients work synergistically, one with another, to provide energy and the raw materials for the repair and maintenance of every cell, organ, gland and fluid in the body. There are, however, certain nutrients, which, as outlined here, do play a particularly focal role in contributing to the good condition and appearance of the skin.

VITAMINS

VITAMIN A (RETINOL AND CAROTENE)

Not for nothing has vitamin A been dubbed 'the skin vitamin'. Adequate supplies are needed principally to ensure healthy eyes and normal low-light vision, but also for the growth and repair of the epidermal tissues as well as the epithelial tissues – the body's 'inner skin' – lining the mouth, nose, ears, eyes, and the respiratory, urinary and genital passages, protecting against invasion by bacteria.

A so-called 'fat-soluble' vitamin, like vitamins D, E and K, vitamin A controls the process of keratinization, the rate and degree at which skin cells are shed and replaced by new ones travelling upwards from the basal layer to the surface, or stratum corneum. Shortage of vitamin A is known to interfere with normal cell turnover. This may lead to a defect known as hyperkeratosis whereby new cells pushing their way upwards from the basal layer die off before they reach the surface, causing a steady build-up of dead flaky tissue, eventually combining with other accumulated surface debris and secretions to clog up the oil sacs and follicles. In turn, this blockage prevents the free-flow of skin oils, eventually leading to pimples, acne, dandruff or a scaly scalp, as well as more serious skin disorders. Conjunctivitis, styes and itching, burning eyes and oversensitivity to light are other common symptoms of vitamin A deficiency. At its most extreme, severe hyperkeratosis is one of the principal factors associated with rough, red, scaly patches of skin common in psoriasis.

Together with vitamin E, vitamin A has been found to increase the permeability of the tiny blood vessels that carry oxygen and nutrients to the cells. By helping to increase the amount of iron carried by the blood, the vitamin also helps to counteract anaemia. Adequate amounts of zinc, however, must be present in the body before vitamin A can be released from the liver into the bloodstream. Both vitamin A and zinc work together to promote the healing of wounds, burns and other forms of skin damage by promoting collagen synthesis. Tests carried out at the University of California show that when vitamin A is applied directly to skin lesions, the condition heals up within a few days.

Relatively few people nowadays risk becoming deficient in vitamin A. It can be derived either from fish liver oils (ie cod), liver, egg yolks, butter, full-fat milk or vegetable sources, including dandelion leaves, carrots, parsley, broccoli and other dark green leafy vegetables which contain large quantities of beta-carotene, or pro-vitamin A, which is converted into vitamin A in the liver. Beta-carotene is the yellowish pigment that gives oranges, melons, carrots, marrows, peaches, etc, their colour. The darker the plant the higher the concentration of carotene, a prime source of vitamin A for anyone eating little or no dairy produce, offal or oily fish. Certain people, such as diabetics, may, however, have difficulty in converting carotene into vitamin A.

Studies suggest that taking more of the pro-vitamin may help reduce sensitivity to ultraviolet light and so protect the skin from some of the damage caused by sunlight, both by stimulating the production of melanin and deactivating harmful free radicals which contribute to premature ageing of the skin. Although vitamin A in large quantities is potentially hazardous, its precursor, beta-carotene, carries no known adverse side-effects if taken in large amounts over a limited period, such as prior to a holiday in the sun. Growing recognition of the relationship between vitamin A and skin healing has led scientists to isolate less synthetic vitamin A compounds known as oral retinoids which are currently proving successful in the treatment of acne and psoriasis. Applied topically, retinoic acid has been found to improve acne as well as reduce symptoms of sun damage and premature ageing, but its possible side-effects (see page 28) must be taken into account.

VITAMIN B COMPLEX

The most heterogeneous of all the vitamin compounds, the B complex group comprises no less than 13 different inter-related components, each one with its own particular role to perform in maintaining health. Although all members of the B group work together to strengthen the nervous system and brain function, to maintain digestive processes and build healthy skin, there are specific ones which appear to be more closely associated with skin maintenance. Water soluble, and therefore derived principally from food as they cannot be stored in the body, B complex vitamins are most likely to be lacking when the body, and the nervous system in particular, are under prolonged assault from stress and toxic substances (ie alcohol or drugs), accounting for numerous skin-related complaints.

VITAMIN B₁ (THIAMIN) was the first of the B vitamins to be discovered. It plays a key role in the conversion of starches and sugars into energy. Healthy brain, nerve and muscle function are directly dependent on adequate amounts of B_1, which is needed in greater amounts during pregnancy, breast feeding, or any digestive, or liver disturbance. Drinking large quantities of alcohol, smoking cigarettes and eating a diet high in sugar, coffee or tea, all interfere with the body's use of thiamin. At its most extreme, severe B_1 deficiency, known as beri-beri, results in muscle wastage, nerve damage and excessive fluid retention. Although rare in developed countries, milder forms of B_1 deficiency may show up as numbness and tingling of the feet and hands, tenderness of the calf muscles, impaired memory and concentration, irritability and depression, night sweats and reduced pain tolerance. The greater the intake of starches and sugars, the higher the need for B_1, found in large amounts in brewers' yeast, wheatgerm, all unprocessed cereals, peas, beans, lentils and brown rice.

VITAMIN B₂ (RIBOFLAVIN) plays a key role in the metabolism of proteins, fats and carbohydrates, aiding the transport of oxygen to the tissues. Deficiency symptoms include cracks around the corners of the mouth, dryness and burning of the lips, eyelids and tongue, and outbreaks of red, greasy and scaly patches similar to dermatitis or eczema, particularly around the sides of the nose. Vertical lip wrinkles that cut into the upper lip are also believed to be due in part to B_2 deficiency, as are oily hair and a sensation of 'burning feet'. Nervous symptoms include dizziness, muscular weakness and shaking. Extra quantities of B_2 may be required during pregnancy and breast feeding, while taking a contraceptive pill, or hormone replacement therapy (HRT) for the menopause, or as a result of consuming moderate to large amounts of alcohol. Principal sources of B_2 are milk and other dairy produce, cereals, liver, lean meat, fish and green leafy vegetables.

VITAMIN B₃ (NIACIN) works in much the same way as B_2 to assist the breakdown and utilization of fats, proteins and carbohydrates in the body and maintain a healthy circulation. The classic symptom of severe B_3 deficiency is pellagra, from the Italian *pelle agra* meaning, literally, 'rough skin'. Pellagra involves scaling, roughness and discoloration resembling sunburn, and other degenerative changes of the skin on the neck, face, hands, lips and tongue, accompanied by diarrhoea and psychological changes including depression, irritability and nervous tension. The skin may become more reactive to sunlight, becoming hyper-pigmented, scaly and raw. Unlike most of the vitamins in the B group which can only be obtained from the diet, B_3 can be manufactured by the body in small quantities via the conversion of an amino acid, tryptophan (one of the constituents of protein), but only when protein and vitamins B_6 and B_2 are also present in large quantities in the diet. Taking certain drugs, such as antibiotics, or drinking a lot of alcohol, may cause a niacin deficiency. The best sources are beef, milk, fish, brewers' yeast, peanuts, whole grains and green leafy vegetables.

VITAMIN B_6 (PYRIDOXINE) has a prime function in helping the body to metabolize protein and fats. Anyone eating a diet composed predominantly of protein stands a greater chance of developing a B_6 deficiency. The vitamin is involved in numerous biochemical processes, principally the maintenance and development of the nervous system, the conversion of tryptophan into vitamin B_3, and the metabolism of magnesium, zinc and essential fatty acids which play an important role in combating inflammatory disorders and skin diseases. Vitamin B_6 is also crucial in regulating the balance between potassium and sodium. Its importance in helping the formation of healthy teeth, gums, skin and blood vessels is well documented and research indicates that the body's requirements of B_6 go up significantly during pregnancy, breast feeding or premenstrual tension, while taking the contraceptive pill, undergoing hormone replacement therapy (HRT) or antibiotic therapy, and during times of stress, low calorie intake or high alcohol consumption. Symptoms of a 'pyridoxine debt' include irritability, nervousness, insomnia, tiredness and depression. These may be accompanied by dandruff, scaliness, flaking or greasiness of the scalp and acne-like rashes especially around the nose, mouth, eyes and over the forehead – symptoms closely resembling B_2 deficiency. The best sources of B_6 are fish, wheatgerm, brewers' yeast, offal, milk, eggs, whole grain cereals, bananas, avocados, nuts, seeds, carrots and some green leafy vegetables. Levels of this vitamin in particular are quickly and easily destroyed through cooking and exposure to light.

VITAMIN B_{12} (CYANOCOBALAMIN) is the only vitamin to contain a mineral element, cobalt. Though only needed by the body in very tiny amounts, the presence of vitamin B_{12} is crucial in counteracting pernicious anaemia and nervous disease. In the absence of B_{12} the stomach is unable to produce an enzyme known as the 'intrinsic factor', vital for the manufacture of new blood cells. Extreme pallor of the skin and mucous membranes, a raw ulcerated tongue, loss of appetite, impaired memory, hair loss and fatigue are inevitable symptoms of B_{12} deficiency. Unlike other B complex vitamins, B_{12} can be stored in the body, principally in the liver, and is also believed to pass into the body via certain forms of bacteria that reside in the intestines. B_{12} deficiency tends to be rare because body stores can last up to five or six years. Certain stomach or intestinal disorders, including insufficient secretions of hydrochloric acid, however, may eventually reduce levels by blocking the absorption of B_{12} from food, allowing deficiency symptoms to creep up slowly yet steadily. The best sources of B_{12} are liver and other organ meats, meat, and to a lesser extent fish, dairy produce, eggs and brewers' yeast – which explains why vegans and vegetarians who eat only vegetables and grains may risk developing eventual B_{12} deficiency.

VITAMIN B_9 (FOLIC ACID) works closely with B_{12} to manufacture normal red blood cells and is therefore crucial to the healthy upkeep of the nervous system. Absorbed from the diet via the first part of the small intestine, folic acid is then stored in the liver. Reserves are usually maintained for up to three or six months. Because sources of folic acid – its name comes, appropriately, from the Latin *folium*, meaning leaf – are limited largely to green vegetables, whole grain cereals, liver and kidneys, minor deficiencies have been found to be relatively widespread although only severe, fullblown deficiencies are likely to lead to iron-deficiency anaemia. Chloasma (mottled hyperpigmentation) which can occur during pregnancy or while taking the contraceptive pill, has been attributed to folic acid deficiency. Folic acid requirements are most likely to rise during times of increased growth, stress and pregnancy (folic acid deficiency has been linked to spina bifida and other congenital neural tube defects), breast feeding and in women taking the contraceptive pill. Green leafy vegetables, such as spinach, greens, etc, offer by far the richest and most readily absorbed source and these should be eaten raw or very lightly cooked to minimize destruction of the vitamin. Brewers' yeast, whole grain cereals, eggs, kidneys and liver are the next best sources.

PANTOTHENIC ACID is a fairly recently discovered member of the B group of vitamins and is widely found in most natural foods. Deficiencies appear to be rare, except amongst people eating mainly refined, processed foods, but requirements are believed to increase, as with all the B vitamins, during times of stress, largely because the function of the adrenal glands which produce the body's main quota of stress hormones, is highly dependent on pantothenic acid. Animal studies also suggest that symptoms of ageing, greying hair, skin deterioration and arthritis, are accelerated when there is insufficient pantothenic acid in the diet. The best

sources are liver, blackstrap molasses, soya beans, brewers'
yeast, eggs and fresh vegetables.

PABA (PARA-AMINO-BENZOIC-ACID) is a vitamin usually classi-
fied as an individual nutrient, although technically it is a component
of folic acid. Its chief claim to fame lies both in its much publicized
alleged power to reverse or prevent greying of the hair as well as its
effectiveness as a sunscreening agent when incorporated in cosmetics. Taking extra quantities of PABA-rich foods – brewers' yeast,
molasses, whole grains – may help reduce the likelihood of sunburn
in people with sensitive skin. Deficiency states are undocumented in
humans but animal research has shown that dermatitis results
when PABA is absent from the diet. In humans, PABA-based skin
ointments appear to be effective in reducing eczema.

BIOTIN deficiencies are also rare, again because of its widespread
distribution in meat, dairy produce and whole grain cereals. Animal studies suggest that a deficiency may cause scaly dermatitis,
hair loss, weakness and tiredness – but these are more likely to
indicate an overall B complex deficiency than simply a shortage of
any one individual component of the group. Longterm antibiotic or
sulphonamide drug therapy, or eating large quantities of raw egg
whites (egg whites contain a protein called avodin which binds
with biotin making it unavailable for absorption), may increase
need for this nutrient. Biotin levels have also been found to be
lower amongst athletes.

CHOLINE is, along with another B vitamin, *inositol*, a key constituent of lecithin, a dietary fat believed to help in the regulation of
blood cholesterol. Choline also contributes to normal muscle function and healthy nerve tissue. Deficiencies are unlikely and the
principal sources are eggs, liver, kidneys, wheatgerm and
brewers' yeast.

A WORD OF CAUTION The roles of all vitamins of the B group are
closely interdependent. Single B vitamin deficiencies are
uncommon and if you are deficient in or more than usually dependent on one of the B group, say because of stress or medication, then
the likelihood is that levels of the others are also low. The best plan,
therefore, is to eat more of those foods which represent the richest
source of all of the B complex vitamins – dairy produce, whole
grains, pulses, green vegetables, offal, wheatgerm, blackstrap
molasses, brewers' yeast and nuts. Although the B complex vitamins cannot build up in the system because they are water soluble,
and therefore rapidly excreted, taking too much of one particular
vitamin in supplement form is usually counter-productive as it may

unbalance the levels of all the others, causing subsequent health problems.

VITAMIN C (ASCORBIC ACID)

No other vitamin holds such a prominent and well-documented position in the annals of food research as vitamin C. Of all individual nutrients, vitamin C is the one most directly and inextricably linked to skin repair and maintenance, and must be present in sufficient quantities in the connective tissue for the formation of collagen, the principal body protein. Without adequate amounts of vitamin C, the structure of the connective tissues begins to break down with the result that wounds heal more slowly and imperfectly, and skin begins to sag and crease, becoming increasingly dry and chapped. Longterm deficiency causes bleeding tissues and gums, loose teeth, loss of hair, haemorrhaging beneath the skin's surface and a tendency to bruise easily. At their most extreme these represent the classic symptoms of scurvy, one of the oldest deficiency diseases recorded in man, and the scourge of seafaring men in the seventeenth and eighteenth centuries who used to go to sea for months on end without any vitamin C in their diet.

Vitamin C also plays an important role in helping the body ward off infection, and it can help the absorption of significantly larger quantities of iron from the diet, thereby providing partial protection against anaemia. Unlike most other mammals, man is unable to synthesize vitamin C, therefore adequate amounts must be present in the diet, particularly during times of stress and illness, especially infection, when the vitamin is utilized by the body in greater quantities. Studies show that those most in need of extra amounts of vitamin C (where therefore supplements may prove useful) are people who smoke, live and work in very polluted atmospheres, or drink large quantities of alcohol, since vitamin C is a powerful anti-oxidant and diuretic and is needed to neutralize toxic substances and eliminate them rapidly from the system. In addition, any skin lesions, including leg ulcers, cold sores, burns, wounds, cuts or post-operative incisions, automatically increase the need for the vitamin as an aid to prompt collagen synthesis.

The richest source of vitamin C are most citrus fruits: oranges, lemons, grapefruit, limes, blackberries, kiwi fruit, rosehips and guavas, and vegetables such as broccoli, peppers, cabbage, with valuable amounts contributed by potatoes. As vitamin C is a water-soluble vitamin, it is virtually impossible to suffer toxic ill effects from taking extra high doses, but large doses can lead to diarrhoea and an increased risk of forming kidney stones. Many doctors believe, however, that the UK recommended daily allowance of

30 g a day is far too low, bearing in mind the limitations of many people's diet, and the numerous factors, such as stress, smoking, drinking, medication and dieting, that increase the body's need for vitamin C. Aiming for levels of about 150 mg per day coming from a diet high in fresh fruit and vegetables, is likely to be an optimum amount for anyone wishing to stay fit and healthy and cultivate the appearance of their skin.

VITAMIN D

Commonly known as the sunshine vitamin, vitamin D is synthesized naturally in the skin, as a result of ultraviolet light stimulus. The darker the skin, the lower the rate of synthesis. It is thought that one of the reasons why white skin develops a tan when exposed to sunlight is to protect the body against the production of dangerously toxic levels of vitamin D, which can prove tremendously harmful if allowed to build up in the system. Similarly, black people, by virtue of their pigmentation, are protected from over-manufacturing vitamin D as a result of being continuously exposed to very intense sunlight.

The chief action of vitamin D is to facilitate calcium metabolism, and so help build and maintain healthy bones and teeth. Any deficiency, therefore – usually due, as described earlier, to insufficient exposure to natural daylight or a diet lacking in oily fish and dairy produce – may result in soft, deformed and weak bones, especially in children (ie rickets), as well as aches and pains in the joints and muscle weakness. Impaired muscle tone inevitably affects the quality of surface facial and body tissues. Like vitamins C and A, D also stimulates the healing of skin tissue, hence the popularity of cod liver oil, the richest source of both vitamins D and A, as a therapeutic additive in ointments and creams used to treat ulcers, sores, cuts and burns.

A diet high in Vitamin D-rich fish oils may also help to improve skin dryness and psoriasis, though this is thought to be due also to the presence of certain essential fatty acids which play an important part in regulating numerous bio-chemical processes and maintaining healthy tissues. In Canada, studies into the effects of these fatty acids on psoriasis indicate that putting patients on a diet supplemented with fish oils produces about 25 per cent improvement in the condition of the skin. A diet that includes a variety of oily fish, including mackerel, salmon, herring, sardines or small quantities of cod liver oil taken as a daily supplement, is likely to provide adequate levels of these essential fatty acids as well as of vitamin D.

VITAMIN E

Touted variously as the anti-ageing, fertility, anti-heart attack or virility vitamin, the protective benefits of vitamin E are believed to lie chiefly in its anti-oxidant properties. In skin, oxidation shows up eventually in the form of mottled pigmentation, crêpiness, wrinkles and brown 'age spots' on the back of the hands. By reducing the amount of oxygen that is needed by the muscles for the normal ongoing processes of oxidation, vitamin E can help to cut down the amount of potential damage wrought by peroxides and other toxic by-products upon individual cells. In particular, vitamin E seems to protect the fat-like structure of the outer cell 'envelope' from being attacked and broken down by peroxides and free radicals, thereby helping the cells maintain their proper function. As more becomes known about the important and protective role played by the essential fatty acids (EFAs) in body chemistry and in the lipid structure of cell membranes, the more valuable appears to be the role of vitamin E in protecting EFAs from oxidation damage.

In addition, vitamin E also widens the blood vessels and boosts the circulation and supply of blood to the tissues, aiding repair and cell synthesis. It actively inhibits the formation of leukotrienes, potent hormone-like substances which form naturally in the bloodstream and which may exacerbate inflammation. By acting in many ways rather like a natural preservative, vitamin E seems to prolong the youthful quality and appearance of all the body tissues, including skin. When applied topically to wounds and burns, the active ingredient in vitamin E oil, alpha tocopherol, has been found to accelerate healing by promoting the flow of blood to the area, also preventing the formation of raised keloid scars.

Vitamin E is also thought to help the body metabolize and utilize vitamin A more effectively. Since vitamin E and iron are mutually incompatible, large quantities of iron in the diet may lower levels of the vitamin, especially in the case of 'iron-enriched' white bread and cereals. Vitamin E is destroyed in the process of acting as an anti-oxidant in the tissues, so the body's need for it goes up whenever there is a greater likelihood of oxidation, for example as a result of eating a diet high in animal fats, sugar and refined foods, smoking and drinking alcohol, stress, exposure to strong sunlight, or medication. It works in close conjunction with vitamin C and selenium, and sufficient quantities of all three nutrients must be present in order to ensure the proper function of one of the body's protective enzymes, glutahione peroxidase, responsible for neutralizing harmful free radicals.

Extra intake of vitamin E, along with vitamin C and zinc, may also help pregnant women avoid getting stretch marks by maintaining a healthy supply of oxygen-rich blood to the tissues. Although vitamin E deficiency is highly unlikely in anyone who eats a well-balanced diet, extra quantities of E-rich foods are advisable for anyone keen to protect their skin from the effects of ageing. The vitamin is present in most cold-pressed polyunsaturated oils and in wheatgerm, whole grain cereals, eggs and green vegetables.

MINERALS

Like vitamins, minerals are a large group of substances vital to normal healthy life. Ranging from the major elements, like calcium and magnesium, to the so-called trace elements, such as zinc and iron, present in very small quantities in the body, all play an important contributory role in combating illness and maintaining healthy organs, tissues and bones, and ensuring normal hormone production and brain, nerve and muscle function. Like vitamins, most major and minor minerals act synergistically – and frequently in close association with certain vitamins – to promote many biological processes.

CALCIUM

Calcium is essential for the formation of strong bones (99 per cent of calcium intake goes towards the upkeep of bones and teeth), healthy nerve tissue, muscle tone and blood clotting. Deficiency may occur as a result of eating a diet low in milk and other milk-based products, or one which is high in bran. The phytates in bran bind up with calcium causing it to become unabsorbable. Insufficient vitamin D synthesis and lowered oestrogen production, for example due to the menopause, or a complete hysterectomy, also directly limit the amount of calcium absorbed by the body. Those with allergies, including eczema, related to cow's milk products, may run a particular risk of becoming calcium deficient and might therefore need to make good the deficit by taking nutritional supplements.

PHOSPHORUS

The mineral works in conjunction with calcium to form bones and teeth. It is widely available in many foods and deficiencies are rare. However, eating large quantities of phosphorus-enriched processed foods and soft drinks can unbalance other mineral levels, for example calcium and zinc. On the other hand, pregnancy, alcoholism, vitamin D deficiency and use of barbiturates or antacids can reduce the amount of phosphorus in the body, so increasing susceptibility to infection and anaemia.

POTASSIUM

Stored in concentration within every cell of the body, potassium is essential for the healthy working of the heart, muscles and nervous system and the maintenance of optimum blood glucose levels. A proper balance of salt and potassium is necessary for good health, especially correct fluid balance. Potassium deficiency, which may occur through eating too much salt, dieting, or from taking diuretics or laxatives which flush both sodium and potassium out of the body, can result in tissue swelling (this may also occur as a result of hormonal changes during the PMT syndrome), weakness, headache, fatigue and depression. Principal dietary sources are mushrooms, bananas, dried dates, wheatgerm, brewers' yeast, asparagus, orange juice and Brussels sprouts.

SODIUM

In the form of salt, sodium is the most common mineral found in foods (and usually incorporated to excess as a hidden additive in processed foods). It is a crucial factor, with potassium, in the regulation of blood pressure and the body's fluid balance. So ubiquitous is salt in the modern diet that the greatest health danger nowadays lies in taking too much rather than too little. In excess, sodium lowers potassium levels, causes fluid retention and raises blood pressure. Anyone suffering from facial puffiness, swollen legs, hands, abdomen, feet or joints, broken red veins or acne rosacea, might be well advised to cut down on salt intake. As iodine can have an irritant action on the tissues, too much iodized salt in the diet can exacerbate spots, pimples and other inflammatory conditions. Deficiencies are rare and result primarily from excessive sweating due to exercise and/ or very hot dry weather, taking too many saunas, vomiting and diarrhoea. Symptoms of lack of sodium include nausea, exhaustion and muscular cramps.

MAGNESIUM

Along with calcium and phosphorus, magnesium is an important component of teeth and bones. Found mostly in nuts, shrimps, soya beans, whole grains and green leafy vegetables, magnesium also regulates many metabolic processes, including the dispersal of sodium, potassium and calcium levels throughout the cell structures, and hence the proper transmission of nerve impulses to the muscles. Deficiencies may occur through dieting, alcoholism or eating too many refined and processed foods. High amounts of bran in the diet also inhibit the absorption of magnesium. Premenstrual discomfort, including irritability, depression and tissue tenderness, may be reduced by taking extra quantities of magnesium along with vitamin B_6.

TRACE ELEMENTS

IRON

Iron is a major component of haemoglobin, the red pigment of blood responsible for carrying oxygen to all body cells. It also contributes to diverse enzyme systems, and maintains the condition of the epithelial tissues. Iron-deficiency anaemia often shows up in ashy, dull facial skin and paleness of the normally bright pink inner eyelid. In addition, the skin beneath the fingernails may fade, creating less contrast against the whiteness of the half moon. Skin lesions, including boils and pimples and generalized itching of the body, are also more likely to occur in people who are anaemic. Tiredness, muscular weakness, giddiness and insomnia are also common side-effects, since anaemia affects all the organs, depriving them of adequate supplies of oxygen.

Low iron status appears to be the most prevalent of all the deficiency states. Women of child-bearing age are particularly susceptible due to monthly blood loss, while drinking excessive alcohol rapidly depletes the body's stores of iron. What is more, iron is notoriously resistant to absorption. Only quite small amounts of the mineral present in food actually pass into the body so it is possible to eat an apparently well-balanced diet yet still risk developing anaemia.

Added to these problems of malabsorption is another factor relative to vegetarians or anyone on a high fibre diet: The phytate present in the bran which is often added to wholemeal bread and breakfast cereals over and above that which is naturally present, further inactivates what iron exists in other foods. However, the presence of an enzyme called phytase, found in all seeds and manufactured by the intestines, is able to counteract the effects of phytic acid. Haem iron, commonly found in meats, is far more easily absorbed and assimilated by the body than the non-haem iron present in green leafy vegetables, pulses and cereals. Coffee taken at mealtimes has also been found to reduce iron absorption from food by as much as 39 per cent. The tannin in tea has a similar, if less dramatically limiting, effect. Conversely, taking vitamin C in the form of fruit juice or fruit during the meal has been shown to bind with non-haem iron and to help carry it across the intestinal lining. A glass of orange juice (containing about 70 mg of vitamin C) pushes up the absorption of iron three-fold. Copper, manganese and cobalt, as well as adequate amounts of protein, vitamin C and B complex vitamins, must also be present to aid iron absorption.

The richest sources of iron are liver, kidneys, heart, egg yolk, blackstrap molasses, shellfish, pulses, seaweed, parsley, red meat and green vegetables. A point worth remembering for anyone trying to stock up on iron is that very high quantities can deplete the levels of zinc in the body – an important element in the maintenance of healthy skin.

COPPER

Involved in the development of brain, nerve and connective tissue, the formation of pigment and the synthesis of haemoglobin, copper deficiencies are unlikely given its widespread presence in water (from copper pipes, copper kettles, containers, etc). Taking high amounts of zinc may, however, cause a copper deficiency. As a toxic substance, too much copper can prove positively harmful. The contraceptive pill elevates blood copper levels, simultaneously reducing zinc levels, while pregnancy may similarly alter the zinc/copper ratio. Prime sources of copper are shellfish (oysters in particular), offal, seeds and prunes.

MANGANESE

An important element in the formation of bone, cartilage, connective tissue and nervous tissue, manganese is necessary for the synthesis of glycoproteins (combined sugars and proteins) in the cells. These glycoproteins form a protective coating around every cell in the body, protecting them against invading viruses – a role similar to that of interferon, another natural anti-viral agent, produced when the body is under attack by harmful viruses. Manganese is crucial for the synthesis of interferon and so contributes to the upkeep of the body's defence systems.

Disorders of the connective tissues, such as arthritis, often go hand in hand with manganese deficiency or an inability of the body to utilize the mineral efficiently. Other diseases, including diabetes, heart and circulatory disorders, have also been associated with low levels of manganese, a mineral which is destroyed through excessive use of chemical fertilizers and is notably absent in over-refined foods. The best natural sources of manganese are sprouted alfalfa seeds, tea (both exceptionally high in manganese), green leafy vegetables and whole grains.

SELENIUM

Also easily destroyed through modern farming methods, selenium works in close partnership with vitamin E to produce the enzyme glutathione peroxidase (GTP), the body's principal anti-oxidant, responsible for preventing and reversing much of the cellular damage caused by oxidation. Since each molecule of GTP contains four atoms of selenium, many bio-chemists regard this mineral as a key component of the body's defence against ageing. It has been found to be 50–100 per cent more effective as an anti-oxidant than vitamin E. Lack of selenium reduces the efficiency of GTP, making body cells more vulnerable to internal pollution and free radical attack. Lack of the enzyme also damages the red cells of the blood, diminishes circulation to the tissues, causing anaemia, while also weakening the ability of the white blood cells to fight infection. Selenium deficiency, therefore, may produce evident changes in skin tissue, such as pallor, infection and hair loss. Good sources of selenium are offal, fish, shellfish, avocados, whole grains, brewers' yeast, garlic, onions and mushrooms. Selenium is also incorporated into special therapeutic shampoos, designed to treat dandruff, ringworm and other sundry surface fungal infections.

SILICON

Found everywhere in nature in microscopic amounts, silicon helps to 'bind' the structure of tissues, so maintaining the strength and elasticity of collagen, elastin, blood vessels, arteries, surface skin, tendons, cartilage and the corneas of the eyes. As part of its job in holding together body tissue, it also helps to keep skin impermeable to liquids and maintains the suppleness of the blood vessel walls. Avocados, buckwheat honey, asparagus, carrots, eggs, lentils, liver and apples are notably rich in silicon.

SULPHUR

Another micro-nutrient that plays a contributory part in collagen synthesis and the formation of red blood cells, sulphur is linked with the functions of the B complex vitamins. It is a prime constituent of keratin, the protein that makes up the stratum corneum, hence its popular name, the 'beauty mineral'. A diet that includes sufficient protein usually supplies ample sulphur. The best sources are eggs, fish, garlic, onion, asparagus, cabbage, dried beans and sprouted beans and seeds.

ZINC

Since zinc forms a crucial element in all growth systems, and is a component of no fewer than 80 body enzymes and hormones, it is little wonder that any deficiency can give rise to diverse health problems. The fact that as much as 20 per cent of body zinc is found in the skin explains why deficiencies may first register in the form of skin disorders and eruptions. Soil levels of the mineral are notoriously prone to depletion through the effects of chemical fertilizers as well as excess rainfall which leaches the mineral out of the soil.

There are numerous instances when deficiency of zinc can occur, for example during pregnancy and lactation, while taking the contraceptive pill, as the result of high protein intake, excess stress or eating a high fibre diet. Bran, in particular, ties up zinc and interferes with its absorption, and other foods, such as cheese, cow's milk, lemons, celery and coffee, have also been found to reduce the body's ability to assimilate zinc efficiently. Drinking large amounts of alcohol leads to zinc deficiency, as does the regular use of diuretics and antibiotic or corticosteroid drug therapy, as well as diseases that affect the kidneys or intestines.

Zinc is vital for the efficient assimilation of the B complex vitamins and assists in the metabolism of essential fatty acids. Healthy nails and skin are dependent on adequate zinc levels, and low levels of zinc in the blood have been widely associated with recurrent acne, boils, psoriasis, dermatitis and weak ridged concave and white-spotted nails, all of which respond well to zinc supplementation in the diet. Wound healing after surgery or an accident is noticeably impaired if there is a zinc shortage.

The body's zinc requirements seem to rise significantly after skin injury – patients recovering from burns have been found to be more prone to excrete zinc, while taking extra amounts often speeds healing. The massive amounts of steroid drugs given to major burn patients cause zinc to be flushed from the system even faster, retarding tissue repair. Some therapists claim that taking extra zinc, vitamin C, B_6 and E during pregnancy may reduce the risk of stretch marks due to the weakening and eventual rupture of collagen and elastin fibres. Essential for proper metabolism of vitamin A, some symptoms of zinc deficiency, like skin scaling and dryness, can masquerade as vitamin A deprivation. There is evidence also that increased vitamin D synthesis enhances the absorption of zinc.

Eating extra quantities of zinc-rich foods at the end of the day may also aid absorption, provided foods that inhibit zinc absorption are avoided at that time. Anyone suffering from wounds or burns, or recovering from surgery, as well as those prone to dermatitis and other chronic skin eruptions – particularly when taking corticosteroid treatment for the condition – should ensure they eat a diet high in zinc-rich foods. These are principally fresh oysters, liver, muscle meats (lamb and beef), ginger root, pecans and other whole nuts, peanut butter, egg yolks, peas, carrots and all whole grains.

IODINE

Iodine has been recognized as an essential trace element for over 150 years. People living in iodine-deficient soil areas are most liable to suffer goitre – enlargement of the thyroid gland. Iodine plays an important part in regulating the manufacture of thyroid hormones which, if upset, can create havoc with any number of biological processes. Excess iodine intake, as a result of eating too much iodized salt or iodine-rich foods, such as clams, shrimps, oysters, haddock, halibut, salmon, sardines, tuna fish, seaweed or dried kelp, or taking certain cough medicines or tonics high in iodine, has been shown to irritate the skin in certain people, as a result of its excretion via the sebaceous glands.

AMINO ACIDS

These rank as the individual building blocks of protein and, after water, constitute the most abundant substance in the body. Although at least 20 amino acids have been identified, the human body can only manufacture 12, which means the rest, the so-called 'essential' amino acids, must be provided by the diet.

Each individual amino acid has a particular role and task to perform within the body. Research is only beginning to yield more precise information as to how these substances operate and interact with other nutrients and bio-chemical substances. Certain amino acids in particular, however, seem to be directly involved in maintaining healthy skin.

Methionine (found in beans, garlic, onions and eggs) is one of the group of sulphur-based amino acids, and is vital for the production of nucleic acid, the regenerative part of the cells and collagen. Together with one of its by-products, *Cysteine* (found mainly in eggs), methionine is important for the proper absorption and assimilation of selenium and contains potent anti-oxidant properties, helping to counter-act the effects of internal pollution.

Cysteine is also an essential component of the immune factor glucathione which, amongst numerous other functions, helps to de-toxify toxic metals (such as lead, mercury and cadmium), alcohol, cigarette smoke, etc, and guard against free radical damage. Cysteine aids metabolism of vitamin B_6 and is found in large quantities in many body proteins, including keratin, the chief constituent of the epidermis, nails and hair.

Lysine, found in grains, nuts and seeds, plays a contributory part in collagen production. It is best known for its ability to control viral infections, in particular herpes simplex.

Tyrosine is a non-essential amino acid, which means that it is formed within the body, rather than being derived from the diet, and is specifically converted from phenylalanine found in nuts, seeds, beans, pulses, meat, fish and milk.

ESSENTIAL FATTY ACIDS (EFAs)

One of the newest, most exciting areas of nutrition research focuses on the protective health benefits of a group of dietary fats known collectively as essential fatty acids (EFAs).

Fatty acids can be divided up quite neatly into the 'good' and the 'bad'. 'Bad' fatty acids are the saturated fatty acids which make up hard fats in meat, butter, lard, etc. 'Good' fatty acids are the polyunsaturated fatty acids (PUFAs) which remain liquid at room temperature and are found principally in vegetable, nut and seed oils, and the monounsaturated fatty acids, which remain liquid but may go cloudy when cold, such as olive oil.

While saturated fats contain potentially harmful triglycerides and, in some cases, large quantities of cholesterol, both of which have been associated with cardiovascular disease and other serious degenerative illnesses, polyunsaturated fatty acids are now increasingly recognized for their beneficial role in promoting health – including that of the skin.

EFAs, so called because they are not synthesized by the body, as is cholesterol, for example, and therefore must come from the food we eat, are essential for bodily functions. EFAs, for instance, form part of the protective lipid barrier, the by-product of skin secretions, on the skin's surface and they also constitute an integral element of the lipid 'envelope' or membrane surrounding every cell in the body.

In terms of positive, health-giving benefits, including the control of skin disease, research has principally centred on two groups of EFAs, known as the Omega-6 and Omega-3 series because of the number of carbon atoms in a particular part of their chemical structure. The prime source of the Omega-6 series is linoleic acid, found mainly in many – though by no means all – polyunsaturated vegetable, nut and seed oils. One of its principal by-products, gamma-linoleic-acid (GLA), which plays a crucial part in maintaining normal metabolic processes, is found only in oil of evening primrose, human breast milk, blackcurrant oil and various herbs such as purslane. The chief source of the Omega-3 series is alpha-linolenic-acid, found in oily fish.

Nutritionists stress that 1 per cent of daily calories should be made up of EFAs, and it would seem that, given the relatively high fat content – often in excess of 40 per cent – of the average Western diet, as well as the increased consumption of polyunsaturated fatty acids in margarines and cooking oils, there should be little danger of any deficiency. Therein lies a supreme paradox. As a result of the complex metabolic function of the different EFAs and their series of metabolites, or by-products, as well as their tendency to be affected by other dietary and health factors, not everyone who has a regular intake of PUFAs automatically obtains their necessary 1 per cent quota of EFAs. In order to understand why, one needs to take a look at the intrinsic structure of certain EFAs, their special functions and the factors which may disrupt those functions.

LINOLEIC ACID (LA) AND GAMMA-LINOLENIC ACID (GLA)

The prime value of EFAs stems from their role as precursors, or forerunners, of other EFAs as well as of a number of short-lived, highly active hormone-like chemicals called prostaglandins and leukotrienes. As far as the skin is concerned, the benefit of EFAs lies in their anti-inflammatory properties as well as in their intrinsic role in maintaining healthy tissue. Lack of linoleic acid (LA) in the diet rapidly leads to dryness and scaling of the skin, increased permeability of the tissues, falling hair, slow or imperfect wound healing, impaired immune function, resulting in infection, and degenerative changes in the collagen and mucopolysaccharide structures – the chemicals that make up intercellular fluid within the connective tissue.

Found chiefly in sunflower, safflower, corn, grapeseed, walnut and wheatgerm oils, linoleic acid is the 'parent' EFA of other Omega-6 fatty acids, including arachidonic acid (although this is also found largely in saturated animal fats), gamma-linolenic acid (GLA) and dihomo-gamma-linolenic acid (DGLA). These metabolic by-products of LA are in turn converted into various prostaglandins of which one in particular, PGE1, specifically controls inflammation, activates T-lymphocytes in the immune system and inhibits abnormal cell turnover (ie hyperkeratinization) which is at the root of many chronic skin disorders. Unfortunately, this conversion process is not always as smoothly efficient as it should be. Numerous factors may impair the enzyme systems necessary for the synthesis of GLA and DGLA, and hence the manufacture of PGE1. The crucial first step in the whole mechanism, the conversion of LA into GLA may prove a disaster area for anyone leading an unhealthy lifestyle.

Certain illnesses, like multiple sclerosis, diabetes, alcoholism, viral infections, or simply eating a diet high in saturated fats, are principally to blame for fouling up the finely tuned conversion system. Dairy produce and meat are a prime source of arachidonic acid, responsible for manufacturing prostaglandins of the so-called '2 series', which promote undesirable inflammatory reactions. Ironically, even a diet that appears healthy because saturated fats have been greatly reduced in favour of polyunsaturated fats, for instance vegetable margarine or vegetable cooking fat, may limit rather than increase EFA intake. This is due to the fact that while perhaps all EFAs consumed are PUFAs, not all PUFAs are EFAs. The process of hydrogenation, or hardening, of natural polyunsaturates accounts for the apparent anomaly. Involving intensive heating, hydrogenation transforms the chemical structure of LA and other 'cis-fatty acids', the form in which they occur in nature, into more stable 'trans-fatty acids', potentially just as harmful to health as saturated fats. Most commercial cooking fats and hard margarines contain anything from 20–50 per cent trans-fatty acids and these fats form the basis of most baked goods and processed foods on the market. Thus, largely destroyed and reconstituted, not only do polyunsaturated oils become devoid of most of their protective benefits, but to all intents and purposes they deprive the body of EFAs, hindering the formation of GLA and

DGLA and interfering with the manufacture of prostaglandins. Therefore, it is advisable to use unrefined (ie, cold-pressed) poly-unsaturated oils and soft margarines.

Since GLA and DGLA are essential elements for prostaglandin synthesis, the obvious answer would be to bypass the potentially imperfect linoleic acid conversion mechanism in the first place. Hence the tremendous popularity of oil of evening primrose as a dietary supplement. Offering the only known ready-made source of GLA, with the exception of human breast milk, because of its ability to promote prostaglandin synthesis as well as reinforce the lipid content of the cell membranes, oil of evening primrose has been found to improve skin dryness as well as combat more serious disorders, notably atopic eczema. In a study conducted at the Bristol Royal Infirmary, reported in the *Lancet* in 1982, nearly 100 patients with atopic eczema showed a significant improvement as a result of taking oil of evening primrose. The precise mode of action as yet appears unclear, although improvement is probably due to increased PGE1 levels which tend to be low in individuals prone to all atopic conditions, including eczema. By boosting T-lymphocyte function, GLA and DGLA further encourage skin healing.

ALPHA-LINOLENIC ACID – THE OMEGA-3 EFAs

The second major group of EFAs belong to the Omega-3 series manufactured from alpha-linolenic acid, long chain highly unsaturated fatty acids which remain most liquid of all at low temperatures and are found in very large quantities in fish oils. Like linoleic acid, alpha-linolenic acid, when absorbed by the body, initiates a complex metabolic chain mechanism, manufacturing eicosapentaenoic acid (EPA) and docosahexaenoic acid (DHA), metabolites which in turn act as precursors of another group of prostaglandins known for their marked anti-inflammatory and anti-thrombotic (ie, anti-blood clotting) properties. Together, the Omega-3s act as an important catalyst in healthy metabolism. Apart from their apparently beneficial action in lowering blood cholesterol, protecting the heart and arteries and maintaining healthy brain tissue, the Omega-3 group of fatty acids also enhances the quality of the skin, slowing down keratinization and speeding up healing.

The skin-healing properties of cod liver oil have been amply documented since the year dot and were traditionally attributed to the high content of vitamins A and D. But now it seems there may be other factors at work. The prostaglandins manufactured from EPA actively reduce the levels of other pro-inflammatory prostaglandins, produced from arachidonic acid, present in meat and dairy produce and synthesized as a metabolite of linoleic acid, especially when there is impaired synthesis of PGE1, which inhibits inflammation. The Omega-3 series therefore appears to exert a calming, healing influence, regulating body chemistry whenever there is a danger of too many pro-inflammatory agents building up in the system, as commonly occurs during allergic reactions, menstrual cramp, migraine or arthritis. For this reason, fish oils are currently in the spotlight for their therapeutic properties in the treatment of rheumatoid arthritis, where inflammation of the joints and tissues becomes especially rampant. EPA and DHA specifically combat the destructive action of groups of potent inflammatory chemicals called leukotrienes which are found in abnormally large quantities in the skin secretions of eczema and psoriasis sufferers. Vitamin E is the only other nutrient known to counteract the effect of leukotrienes.

Recent medical trials into the effects of fish oils on psoriasis show that by acting as an anti-inflammatory agent they help to reduce redness, itching and scaling, while diminishing the number and size of psoriatic plaques on the body. Because of their effectiveness in lowering cholesterol in the blood and strengthening the immune system, fish oils are also recommended to offset some of the potentially harmful side-effects of certain drugs, including corticosteroids, retinoic acid and PUVA therapy (strong ultraviolet light radiation used in conjunction with skin photosensitizing drugs), increasingly prescribed to treat psoriasis, vitiligo, acne and eczema.

Scientists researching the therapeutic potential of EPA and DHA believe that anyone with a tendency to inflammatory disorders, including skin diseases like psoriasis and eczema, should not only limit the amount of animal and dairy fat in the diet but also reduce the intake of polyunsaturated plant oils, especially the processed variety high in trans-fatty acids. The common 'bogey' in all of these is arachidonic acid, the precursor of pro-inflammatory prostaglandins and leukotrienes, which is in perpetual competition with EPA and DHA, in a bid to become assimilated and further converted into either welcome or unwelcome by-products. Theoretically at any rate, the greater the intake of EPA and DHA, the lesser the likelihood of excess arachidonic acid 'taking over' the system. Increasing the amount of oily fish eaten, and perhaps using cod liver oil as a supplement may therefore help in promoting a healthy heart, arteries, brain function and joints, as well as warding off skin disorders, largely by balancing the levels of biochemical components in the blood and tissues.

IN THE RAW

For optimum health as well as good-looking skin there can be no substitute for a diet which includes a large variety of wholesome, unprocessed foods, such as fresh vegetables, salads, fruit, pulses, seeds, nuts and whole grain cereals, providing the richest source of vitamins, minerals, trace elements, amino acids and enzymes. However, the food we eat is in constant danger of becoming depleted of many of its vital health-giving constituents. Although this applies particularly to processed foods, even with fresh crops, to all intents and purposes chock-full of nutrients, a certain amount of depletion often seems inevitable, beginning sometimes, quite literally, at grassroots level.

Many of today's mass-produced crops, intensively grown with the aid of powerful chemical fertilizers, are deprived of many essential minerals already stripped from the soil or else present only in very small quantities. Fruit, often grown under artificial conditions, or harvested while unripe and then artificially ripened, sometimes even injected with colourants, is unable, through insufficient ultraviolet light stimulus, to synthesize its full quota of vitamins. Levels of the all-important yet highly vulnerable B complex vitamins, vitamin C and the trace elements are prone to diminish during long periods of storage and exposure to light and heat. The final insult, however, occurs in the kitchen when a large proportion of the remaining nutrients is effectively destroyed through overcooking.

Foods that are most nutrient-dense are inevitably those which should be cooked very lightly and for brief periods. For example, steaming and quick stir-frying are the two methods likely to ensure preservation of the greatest proportion of nutrients in vegetables. Nutritionally richer by far, however, are those that are eaten raw.

The positive benefits of following a diet composed partly or very largely of raw foods, especially vegetables, fruit, seeds, nuts and grains, are infinite and likely to be reflected in improved skin tone and texture. Raw vegetables and many fruits, if eaten with their skins, provide an excellent natural source of roughage, acting as an 'intestinal broom' to help eliminate waste matter, cleanse the colon, purify the bloodstream and strengthen the function of the bowels, kidneys and intestines. A salads-only regime or a 100 per cent raw vegetable and fruit diet, supplemented with juice extracts, lasting anything from three to fourteen days may work wonders in helping to refine the skin, eliminate spots, blemishes and sallowness and add a fresh glow to the complexion.

All vegetables and many fruits are alkaline in composition and can therefore help to maintain the natural alkalinity of the blood.

In a healthy body, the proportion of alkaline salts is 80 per cent, or four to one. Modern living has a tendency however to upset this balance, with often far-reaching adverse side-effects. Meat, dairy produce, sweets, tea, coffee, alcohol, and all processed foods are predominantly high acid-forming foods which, especially if consumed in excess, not only cause internal pollution and cross-linking due to oxidation and the formation of free radicals, but may produce over-acidity, a contributory factor in many inflammatory and degenerative diseases, such as ulcers, gout, arthritis and eczema.

Protein and animal fats also take time and extra energy to become fully digested, and, if eaten in very high quantities, may eventually tax and weaken the digestive organs. The therapeutic value of such time-honoured natural remedies as fasting, drinking only fruit juice or herbal teas, or eating only raw vegetables, is believed to be due largely to the healing and regenerative processes of these vital organs which can only come properly into play when the system is not constantly overloaded with hard-to-digest protein, fat and high acid-forming foods.

ENZYMES – NATURE'S CATALYSTS

Apart from providing the richest possible source of necessary vitamins, minerals and fibre, as well as vegetable protein (which is more easily assimilated and, provided foods are varied and balanced, just as nutritious as animal protein), raw food also contains certain enzymes that work in conjunction with the body's own digestive enzymes to ensure normal, healthy metabolism. Without the presence of many different enzymes in the body, acting as catalysts at every stage of the digestion and absorption of nutrients, normal biological processes could not take place and the human mechanism would fail.

The principal action of enzymes, after helping in the breakdown and assimilation of food, is to aid the process of tissue repair and cell regeneration, and to boost the production of protective bacteria in the colon and intestines, which is vital to the proper function of the immune system. Enzymes therefore guard against infections linked to altered microflora on the mucous membranes, for instance thrush or chronic candidiasis. Skin disorders linked to candidiasis can take numerous forms, including itching, hives, allergic dermatitis and fungal nail or skin infections. These normally protective gut bacteria are particularly prone to destruction by certain drugs, such as antibiotics, the contraceptive pill and corticosteroids; the chemicals found in meat and dairy produce (ie, antibiotics and hormones); the effects of stress and a diet high in processed foods, animal protein, sugar, fats and spices.

Since they are living, heat-sensitive substances, the so-called proteolytic (protein-digesting) enzymes in raw food, which do much to boost the function of the body's enzymes, especially where there is an imbalance or deficiency, are easily destroyed during cooking. At temperatures below 50°C (122°F) they may be partially preserved, but if vegetables are boiled or deep-frozen after blanching, or canned, their enzyme content is rapidly reduced to nil. Fresh fruit and their juices, freshly chopped or shredded vegetables, uncooked fresh nuts, seeds (including sunflower, sesame and pumpkin) and sprouted grains, beans and seeds, including alfalfa (although no more than 25 g/l oz alfalfa sprouts should be eaten per day as excess intakes have been linked to an inflammatory disease, systemic lupus erythematosis), wheat, mung beans, chick-peas, soya beans and lentils, all contain a particularly rich cache of B complex vitamins, vitamin C, enzymes and trace elements. It has been estimated that sunflower seeds, when compared to the same amount of steak, contain 25 times more vitamin B_1, 3½ times more iron, twice the level of protein and large amounts of vitamin E. Sprouting seeds, grains and pulses multiplies their content of vitamins A, B complex, C and E by up to 700 per cent. Sprouting also neutralizes the phytates normally present in beans and seeds which largely inhibit the absorption of important nutrients such as zinc and calcium.

Some tropical fruits, such as papayas, mangoes and pineapples, contain notably high quantities of enzymes recognized for their ability to dissolve defective, cross-linked protein. Some researchers into ageing believe that these substances may also help to reverse some of the ill effects of oxidation on skin tissue, including hardened, cross-linked collagen. The anti-inflammatory skin- and tissue-healing properties of papaya, when applied externally, have been in part credited to the power of its natural enzyme, papain. To derive the optimal concentrated effects of these enzymes, the fruit should ideally be eaten on its own and on an empty stomach.

ALLERGIES

Eczema, which is estimated to affect 1–3 per cent of the population, often occurs early on in childhood and sufferers may frequently be susceptible to other atopic disorders such as hay fever, migraine and asthma. Childhood eczema often improves or disappears altogether prior to or at puberty, yet certain individuals may only develop the disorder once they grow up, sometimes becoming overly dependent on certain foods to which they are increasingly, yet unknowingly, sensitized. Although the substances, both environmental and/or dietary, that trigger or exacerbate the redness, blistering, itching, scaling, swelling and raw skin may be numerous, the most common dietary allergens tend to be cow's milk and cow's milk products, eggs and wheat products, followed by meat (especially pork), shellfish and fish, nuts and chocolate. These may be implicated in chronic, severe eczema or in sudden eruptions of hives (nettle rash) which generally last no more than about 24 hours. Hives is also more likely to result from eating food that does not normally feature in the everyday diet, for example strawberries or shellfish.

THE DETECTIVE WORK

The first step in nailing down any single substance or group of food allergens is to follow a strict exclusion diet whereby certain categories of foods, for example milk and dairy produce, types of meat, etc, are eliminated completely for about two weeks, then reintroduced in order to establish whether or not there is any adverse reaction. During this period it is important to keep a diary listing all foods consumed and eliminated, down to the last detail, and to record all relevant skin symptoms.

Some allergens or irritants, however, do not readily reveal their identity and may prove fiendishly hard to trace. Certain people with highly sensitive skin and a predisposition to either eczema, acne rosacea or psoriasis may react adversely to certain 'hidden' taste enhancers used in large quantities in processed and preserved foods. By sticking very largely to fresh unprocessed fare, it is possible to avoid such unwelcome ingredients altogether.

The same principle of avoidance applies to additives, the 20th century scourge of anyone with a sensitive allergy-prone skin or physical disposition. An allergy or skin sensitivity may be linked to just one or two additives, but the job of tracking down the offending substance may involve a period of all-out detective work. With literally many dozens of artificial colouring agents and preservatives now in use by the food industry for inclusion in foods and beverages of every type, isolating those chemicals responsible for causing an irritant or allergic reaction is no mean feat. Since as yet not all manufacturers include a complete specific list of ingredients on the packaging, the task can ultimately prove frustrating and time-consuming in the extreme. The most common E additives, however, known to be associated with allergic reactions, including skin rashes, are the azo (coaltar) dyes (E102–110 and E122–133) – which include tartrazine (E102), quinoline yellow (E104), carmosine (E122), erythrosine (E127) and indigo carmine (E132)

– and preservatives such as benzoates (E210–219) and meta-bisulphites (E220–227). If in doubt, wherever a fresh, chemically uncontaminated alternative to processed food exists, try to opt for that instead, especially if allergies and rashes are a persistent and recurrent problem.

PLANT POWER

Fasting and the consumption of herbal teas, infusions or extracts to detoxify the system and speed the body's own healing action is an age-old remedy amply documented in all the annals of nature cure, ancient and modern. There is little doubt that, providing you are in good health, spending a few days eating little or no food, and drinking lemon juice or herbal infusions only, can help to increase energy, combat infection, improve the circulation, and counteract such metabolic disorders as acidity, constipation, fluid retention and indigestion, thereby helping to improve the appearance of the skin.

People who fast regularly report that although their skin condition may at first deteriorate, becoming spotty, greasy and blotchy, once the initial fasting period is over, its appearance is significantly brighter, clearer and tauter, as the toxins in the system are completely eliminated. Apart from taking freshly extracted vegetable and/or fruit juices throughout the fast, there are certain plants and herbs that are recognized for their healing, purifying or antibacterial properties.

STINGING NETTLES are rich in vitamin C, iron, chlorophyll and glucoquinone. They have an astringent effect, stimulate metabolism, eliminate uric acid and are recommended for skin disorders. They can be brewed to make tea or pressed to extract juice.

HORSE-TAIL contains silicic acid, saponin and organic acids, and assists natural healing processes. It also has a mild diuretic action.

SOAP-WORT is high in saponins and acts as an expectorant, diuretic and laxative, while stimulating the activity of the skin cells. The root should be shredded, soaked in water, then heated, and the liquid drunk twice daily.

MARIGOLD contains carotenoids, saponin, acids and mucins. It has an anti-inflammatory action and promotes wound healing.

GREAT BURDOCK contains mucilage, acids and antibiotic

substances. It acts as a gentle diuretic and stimulates wound healing.

COMFREY is rich in allantoin and speeds wound healing, promotes the formation of new connective tissue, soothes irritation and inhibits inflammation. It is best drunk as a tisane.

GERMAN CHAMOMILE is high in essential oil with chamazulene and bisabol oil, mucins and fatty acids. It is known for its ability to inhibit inflammation, aid wound healing and combat infection.

ST JOHN'S WORT contains tannin, resin, essential oil and hypercin, which work together to activate the digestive system and assist wound healing.

HEARTSEASE (a member of the pansy family) contains saponins, rutin, some salicylic acid compounds, calcium and magnesium salts and is particularly recommended for clearing skin rashes, including eczema, and outbreaks of spots and pimples. It should be brewed as tea and drunk two or three times a day.

A–Z of Skin Problems

ACNE

COMMON CAUSES | Over-active oil glands due to hormonal imbalance; clogged-up ducts and inflamed follicles lead to pimples, blackheads, cysts and boils.

DIETARY FACTORS | Contrary to popular belief, there is no proven link between diet and spots or acne, although excessive iodized salt or iodine-high foods and medicines may inflame the skin. Too many refined sweet, fatty or spicy foods, high in additives, can also act as an irritant in certain people with allergy-prone skin.

KEY NUTRIENTS | Extra amounts of zinc. If taken as a supplement, no more than 30–40 mg per day taken on its own 1½ hours after eating, preferably at night. Outbreaks of acne linked to PMT or the contraceptive pill may respond to extra intake of zinc and B complex vitamins, especially B_6. Small amounts of selenium (200 mcg per day) seem to improve acne in men.

ACNE ROSACEA

COMMON CAUSES | Chronic allergic hypersensitivity of the skin, especially pronounced in middle age, characterized by heightened facial tone, frequent violent flushing, purplish lumps and bumps beneath the surface, broken red veins on cheeks and nose.

DIETARY FACTORS | Extreme sensitivity to extremes of hot and cold, very hot and spicy or cold food, alcohol and all hot beverages. Certain 'trigger' foods may produce an allergic reaction, dilating and weakening the blood vessels, causing inflammation. Corticosteroid ointments may further damage the skin and weaken its resistance to bacteria.

KEY NUTRIENTS   Extra B complex vitamins, vitamin C, silicon and zinc, to protect the capillary walls, strengthen the immune system and combat infection.

AGEING SKIN (wrinkles, creases, brown blotches and loss of elasticity)

COMMON CAUSES   Too much exposure to strong sunlight, insufficient surface protection (skin cream) against dehydration, cigarette smoking, drinking large amounts of alcohol, use of drugs, longterm illness, longterm corticosteroid ointment therapy, rapid and extreme weight loss, hormonal imbalance (eg low oestrogen) especially during and post menopause.

DIETARY FACTORS   Excessive alcohol consumption and crash dieting leads to nutritional deficiencies, mainly lack of vitamin C, zinc, selenium, amino acids and essential fatty acids.

KEY NUTRIENTS   Increased intake of sulphur-rich foods (eggs, garlic, onion, fish, beans), vitamin C (citrus and other fruits), zinc (offal, seafood, whole nuts, carrots and whole grains), selenium (shellfish, brewers' yeast, cabbage, garlic and onions). Also emphasis on regular intake of EFAs, as in oil of evening primrose and fish oils. Extra vitamin E (wheatgerm, asparagus) may help protect against oxidation.

BOILS AND ABSCESSES

COMMON CAUSES
Infection due to bacteria. Frequent recurrence may be caused by lowered immunity. Iron deficiency further heightens susceptibility to infection.

DIETARY FACTORS
Shortage of B complex vitamins, vitamin C, manganese; too many refined processed foods, high alcohol consumption.

KEY NUTRIENTS
Extra intake of iron (offal, spinach and other dark green vegetables, blackstrap molasses), vitamin C (all fruit), B complex (dairy produce, whole grains, sprouted seeds, grains and pulses, wheatgerm, brewers' yeast), zinc (seafood, whole nuts, peas, liver) and selenium (cabbage, avocados, garlic, onions, shellfish) to speed healing. Extra manganese (whole grains, avocados, nuts) can help to strengthen the body's defence system.

BROKEN RED VEINS

COMMON CAUSES
Most frequently occurs in delicate, sensitive skin, due to impaired circulation (if the problem affects the legs) and congested blood vessels. Fragile capillary walls are prone to dilate and rupture causing blood to seep out in minute quantities into the tissues. Corticosteroid ointments or drugs and high blood pressure may aggravate the problem.

DIETARY FACTORS
Too many salty, spicy foods, alcohol and very hot beverages. Shortage of vitamins C and E, silicon and sulphur-rich foods may also weaken the capillaries.

KEY NUTRIENTS
Extra vitamin C (citrus fruit) and silicon (avocados, buckwheat honey, asparagus, lentils, eggs, apples) to strengthen the

capillary walls; vitamin E (polyunsaturated oils, nuts, whole grains).

BRUISES

COMMON CAUSES   Individuals with very delicate fair skin may be more prone to bruising even as a result of very minor pressure or impact.

DIETARY FACTORS   None, except vitamin C deficiency in very severe cases where brushing is accompanied by bleeding gums and other skin lesions.

KEY NUTRIENTS   Vitamin C (fruit and vegetables), vitamin E (wheatgerm), selenium (garlic, onions and shellfish) and zinc (seafood, liver, whole nuts) to aid tissue healing.

BURNS

COMMON CAUSES   Very hot or scalding fluids or food, fire, corrosive chemicals, sunlight.

DIETARY FACTORS   Any deficiency of vitamin C or zinc may retard the formation of new tissue. Large amounts of vitamin E taken internally and applied externally to the wounds speeds healing and helps prevent scarring. Nutritional supplements may consist of up to 800 IU per day during recovery. Extra protein, zinc, silicon, sulphur, selenium and vitamin C further aid collagen synthesis.

KEY NUTRIENTS   Protein and zinc-rich foods; vitamin C (fruit and vegetables); vitamin E (wheatgerm and other polyunsaturated oils, asparagus and nuts).

CHAPPED AND CRACKED SKIN/LIPS

COMMON CAUSES	Very dry indoor and outdoor atmospheres, strong sunlight, dehydration due to fever, colds, flu and other infections, and cigarette smoking.
DIETARY FACTORS	Deficiency of B complex vitamins, mainly B_6, B_{12} and folic acid – in particular, if severe, a specific shortage of B_2.
KEY NUTRIENTS	Extra foods high in B complex vitamins (whole grain, brewers' yeast), vitamin C (fruit), zinc (seafood, liver, whole nuts) and selenium (shellfish, onions, garlic, cabbage) for healing. Increase consumption of foods high in LA, GLA (polyunsaturated vegetable oils) and EPA (fish oils), and oil of evening primrose.

COLD SORES (Including types 1 and 2 herpes simplex and genitalis)

COMMON CAUSES	Lowered immunity, stress, extremes of temperature, excessive strong sunlight.
DIETARY FACTORS	Lowered immunity may be due to deficiencies of B complex vitamins, vitamin C or selenium.
KEY NUTRIENTS	Extra quantities of manganese (whole grains, avocados, nuts), vitamin C, and the amino acid, lysine (taken as a supplement 300–1200 mg daily), while making sure the diet is low in its 'opposite', arginine (peanuts, chocolate, seeds and cereals) which appears to favour the growth of the herpes simplex virus.

DRYNESS (scaling, itching, surface lines, tautness)

COMMON CAUSES — Dehydration of the epidermis due to environmental extremes, strong sunlight etc; anorexia; rapid weight loss; cigarette smoking; use of diuretics and laxatives; long distance air travel; exposure to VDUs; alcohol consumption; shortage of oestrogen after the menopause.

DIETARY FACTORS — Lack of sufficient vitamin A, vitamin E and insufficient amounts of EFAs are often associated with chronic dryness, a problem linked to eating a vegan or restricted vegetarian diet that contains insufficient protein or dairy produce.

KEY NUTRIENTS — Increased intake of betacarotene (carrots and all other yellow-orange fruit and vegetables), LA (safflower and sunflower oils), GLA (oil of evening primrose), EPA (oily fish), silicon (avocados, asparagus, lentils, eggs, buckwheat honey), sulphur-based amino acids (egg, fish, garlic, dried beans, sprouts), vitamin E (wheatgerm), vitamin C, zinc and selenium.

ECZEMA

COMMON CAUSES — Inflammation can be caused by environmental or dietary allergens due to an inherited defect in normal production of antibodies, often exacerbated by stress or emotional shock.

DIETARY FACTORS — Apart from possible food intolerance in some sufferers, there may be an imbalance of certain chemicals (ie, prostaglandins) in the body because of faulty EFA metabolism. Zinc also appears to be lower in eczema sufferers.

| KEY NUTRIENTS | Extra amounts of GLA (evening primrose oil) EPA and DHA (fish oils) have both proven useful in treating eczema. Extra zinc, selenium and vitamin C may all encourage healing. B complex vitamins help to strengthen the nervous and immune systems. |

EYE IRRITATION OR INFLAMMATION

COMMON CAUSES	Lowered immune function, pollution, VDU 'skin sickness' or allergy to synthetic chemicals.
DIETARY FACTORS	Shortage of vitamin A, essential for normal vision and healthy membrane, and lack of vitamin B_2.
KEY NUTRIENTS	Increased intake of foods high in vitamin A (oily fish, liver, egg yolks, yellow fruit and dark yellow or green vegetables) and B complex vitamins (whole grains, brewers' yeast, etc).

LEG ULCERS

COMMON CAUSES	Often associated with fluid retention, obesity, standing for long periods and inactivity, which may lead to faulty circulation and varicose veins, especially in elderly people.
DIETARY FACTORS	A diet high in refined foods, sugar, animal fats, insufficient fibre, too much salt.
KEY NUTRIENTS	Increased intake of vitamin C and zinc, also vitamin E and selenium, to control infection, accelerate wound healing and improve circulation. Whole grains, pulses, whole fruit and vegetables for extra fibre. Reduced salt intake.

OILY SKIN

COMMON CAUSES — The basic skin type is invariably hereditary, but oiliness may be aggravated through stress, a very hot humid environment or taking the contraceptive pill.

DIETARY FACTORS — Too much alcohol, a diet composed predominantly of very rich, fried fatty foods, sugar and refined carbohydrates (cakes, biscuits, pies, etc) and nuts (high in oil). Oil production may be triggered by certain E additives and 'hidden' spices in packaged food. Seborrhoeic dermatitis – a red greasy itchy rash – can also be caused through vitamin B_6 or B_2 deficiency.

KEY NUTRIENTS — Increased consumption of fruit, fresh – preferably raw where possible – vegetables, salads, whole grains, pulses, sprouted seeds and grains – all high in B complex vitamins and low in fat.

PALLOR/ SALLOWNESS

COMMON CAUSES — Anaemia due to iron deficiency, sometimes linked to vitamin B_{12} or folic acid shortage. Sluggish circulation, inefficient elimination of toxins eventually shows up in muddy facial skin tone.

DIETARY FACTORS — Too many refined and processed foods and insufficient roughage leads to constipation and toxic build-up. A diet low in easily absorbable iron (ie liver) and vitamin C which aids the absorption of iron from plant foods. Large amounts of coffee or tea taken during meals also reduce iron absorption.

KEY NUTRIENTS — Increased intake of offal and dark green vegetables high in iron and folic acid (broccoli, spinach, blackstrap molasses). Take extra vitamin C with meals to raise levels of iron absorbed. Liver and other organ meats are high in both easily absorbable iron and vitamin B_{12}. To improve circulation and assist elimination, eat plenty of raw vegetables, salads and fruit which supply plenty of vitamin C. Drink water or herbal teas to encourage the elimination of toxins. Vitamin E (wheatgerm, etc) boosts circulation of blood.

PSORIASIS

COMMON CAUSES

Red raw scaly patches are usually found on the arms, hands, feet, legs and trunk, but rarely on the face and are thought to be due to hyperkeratinization, a defect in the rate at which new skin cells are formed. The basic underlying causes remain unknown but lowered immunity often linked to stress and emotional trauma may be a contributory factor.

DIETARY FACTORS

As with people suffering from eczema, EFAs may be imperfectly metabolized by the body. A diet high in refined foods, spices, caffeine and alcohol may aggravate the condition in some individuals. Longterm use of corticosteroid ointments can damage the skin even further and lower the immune system.

KEY NUTRIENTS

Extra amounts of EPA and DHA (oily fish, cod liver oil) appear to improve and control the condition. Foods high in zinc (oysters and other shellfish, liver, red meat, cheese, oily fish, wholemeal bread) may aid healing. Vitamin C and the B complex vitamins (whole grains, brewers' yeast, green vegetables, molasses, sprouted grains and seeds, etc) protect the nerves and the immune system.

STRETCH MARKS

COMMON CAUSES   Greatly increased skin tension, especially over the hips, tummy, thighs and breasts, usually due to pregnancy or excessive weight gain, resulting in weakening and eventual rupture of the underlying elastin and collagen fibres responsible for maintaining surface tension and firmness.

DIETARY FACTORS   Any nutritional deficiency during pregnancy may affect skin condition but the damage may be particularly marked when there is a shortage of any of the nutrients specifically needed for connective tissue repair and collagen synthesis – vitamins C, E, zinc and selenium. Once stretch marks have formed, they cannot be removed through diet or external treatment, so the only strategy is prevention in the form of a balanced diet and judicious weight control.

KEY NUTRIENTS   Extra quantities of those nutrients that play a key role in collagen and elastin synthesis: vitamin C (fruit and vegetables), zinc (shellfish, liver, red meat, oily fish), selenium (shellfish, cabbage, garlic, onions, mushrooms), silicon (avocados, asparagus, eggs, lentils, etc). Extra vitamin E taken internally (wheatgerm, etc) and massaged into the skin as a conditioner may also strengthen the elasticity of the tissues and prevent weakening of the underlying fibres.

SUNBURN

COMMON CAUSES   Excessive exposure to very strong sunlight, especially without using an effective sun-screening agent. Reflection from sand, water, snow, glass, concrete, further intensifies the impact of burning rays, which are at their strongest between 11 am and 3 pm. People with fair, freckled skin, reddish hair and blue eyes are most at risk.

DIETARY FACTORS   None – although some researchers believe that impaired synthesis of betacarotene affects melanin production and causes the skin to become more vulnerable.

KEY NUTRIENTS   Proper and effective protection against the sun can only come from without. However, taking extra amounts of betacarotene (carrots and other dark yellow vegetables and fruit), as well as foods high in phenylalanine (nuts, seeds, pulses, meat, fish, dairy produce and fruit) and PABA (brewers' yeast, molasses, whole grains) may help to reduce the vulnerability of people with very delicate skin. Should sunburn occur, increase the intake of zinc, vitamin C and vitamin E (wheatgerm, asparagus) while applying any acidic substance, such as natural yogurt or tomato, immediately to reduce the burn, followed later by vitamin E to accelerate healing.

SWELLING (Oedema)

COMMON CAUSES   Pre-menstrual or menopausal hormone imbalances or impaired kidney function, may commonly lead to fluid retention. Frequent use of diuretics, by upsetting the sodium/potassium balance of the body, can cause a rebound effect, resulting in further fluid gain.

DIETARY FACTORS   Potassium deficiency can lead to excess salt (sodium chloride) levels, a key factor in fluid retention. A diet high in salt, much of it in invisible form in processed foods, may also upset the body's fluid balance.

KEY NUTRIENTS   Increased intake of potassium-rich foods – mushrooms, bananas, dried dates, wheatgerm, brewers' yeast, Brussels sprouts, lentils and prunes. Vitamin B_6 (whole grains, molasses, brewers' yeast) and magnesium (nuts, shrimps, soya beans, green leafy vegetables, whole grains) also help to counteract oedema associated with PMT.

THRUSH
(Candidiasis)

COMMON CAUSES

An imbalance in the protective micro-flora which reside in the gut, often the by-product of taking the contraceptive pill, antibiotics, or being subject to excessive stress. Very humid, warm environments and wearing restrictive clothing may also contribute to the infection. In very severe cases, reduced immunity may result in the spread of more generalized yeast infections including skin rashes and itchiness.

DIETARY FACTORS

Iron and zinc deficiencies are common in immune suppression, a by-product of more serious yeast infection, and those particularly at risk are women on a strict vegetarian or vegan diet. The spread of candidiasis is aggravated in particular by all foods that actively nurture the yeast organism, predominantly refined carbohydrates (white flour, white or brown sugar), yeasted foods (including yeast extract, frozen or concentrated orange juice, cheese, bread made with yeast, alcohol, grapes and grape juice, unpeeled fruit, raisins and sultanas).

KEY NUTRIENTS

Concentrate on eating foods that contain natural anti-fungal properties such as garlic; onions; fresh (raw if possible) green, leafy vegetables; oily fish; live yogurt; sunflower, olive and cold-pressed linseed oils; oil of evening primrose; foods low in carbohydrates. Increased iron- and zinc-rich foods (shellfish and oily fish, liver, kidneys, red meat) further help to boost immune function. Raw sprouted seeds, grains and pulses are also rich in enzymes which help to protect the distribution of micro-flora in the digestive tract.

WOUNDS AND CUTS

COMMON CAUSES

Whether due to accident or surgery the rate of healing and the quality of new tissue, including the non-formation of scars, is determined largely by adequate supplies of oxygen-rich blood and nutrients to the fibroblast cells responsible for collagen synthesis.

DIETARY FACTORS

Excessive alcohol, cigarette smoking, and a diet high in refined processed foods, use of corticosteroids and other drugs, radiation, and chemotherapy may reduce the supply of these nutrients – principally zinc, vitamin C, selenium and vitamin E – to the living tissues, while simultaneously depleting immune function.

KEY NUTRIENTS

To strengthen the immune system and accelerate wound healing, increase the intake of B complex vitamins, vitamin C (citrus fruit as well as extra supplements, 1–3 grams per day); zinc (shellfish, oily fish, liver, red meat, wholemeal bread etc. plus extra supplements, 30–50 mg per day), selenium (garlic, onions, cabbage, shellfish, mushrooms), manganese (whole grains, avocados). Extra vitamin E (wheatgerm, asparagus and nuts, plus extra supplements 400–800 IU per day) taken internally and applied directly to the skin speeds healing while helping prevent scars.

Recipe Analysis and Nutrition Labelling

Each recipe in the following section is accompanied by a nutritional analysis. A serving of each recipe has been computer-analysed for its calorie (kilojoule), protein, fat and carbohydrate content, together with dietary fibre, vitamins and minerals which have been star-rated – the more stars the more of that nutrient is present.

Figures for dietary fibre appear whether it attains star-rating or not. The vitamins and minerals are selected according to the greatest amount present per serving, and those which are particularly beneficial to maintaining a healthy skin are given most prominence.

Star-rating is based on the percentages of Recommended Daily Amounts (RDA) of fibre, vitamins and minerals as follows:

RECOMMENDED DAILY AMOUNTS

The daily amounts of nutrients shown right are those recommended by the Department of Health and Social Security for an 18–34 year old moderately active man. However, those marked with an asterisk(*) are amounts recommended in the United States of America in 1980 for male and female adults. All the recipes have been selected for their contribution of nutrients that help towards maintaining a healthy skin. Taking into account healthy eating recommendations, every attempt has been made to conserve nutrients and increase fibre, while reducing the amounts of fat (particularly saturated fat), processed sugar and salt.

	Protein	=	72 g
	Fibre	=	30 g
	Cholesterol	=	300 mg
	Potassium	=	3048 mg
	Calcium	=	500 mg
	Iron	=	12 mg
*	Magnesium	=	350 mg
*	Phosphorus	=	800 mg
*	Copper	=	2.52 mg
*	Zinc	=	15 mg
	Vitamin A	=	750 mcg
	Thiamin (B_1)	=	1.2 mg
	Riboflavin (B_2)	=	1.6 mg
	Niacin	=	18 mg
*	Vitamin B_6	=	2.2 mg
	Vitamin B_{12}	=	3 mcg
	Folic acid	=	300 mcg
*	Pantothenic acid	=	5.6 mg
*	Biotin	=	150 mcg
	Vitamin C	=	30 mg
*	Vitamin D	=	10 mcg
*	Vitamin E	=	10 mg

NOTE: Due to the varying quality of many fresh foods, these nutrient levels should be regarded as approximate.

PER SERVING

★	10–20%
★ ★	21–40%
★ ★ ★	41–60%
★ ★ ★ ★	61–80%
★ ★ ★ ★ ★	81–100% or more

1

Breakfast and Brunch

Few people nowadays tuck into a big cooked breakfast every morning, preferring something lighter and quicker such as cereal or toast. Luckily, this is a far more healthy idea generally, and the skin in particular will be better off without the extra fat involved in a traditional cooked breakfast. When it comes to brunch, however, a light cooked meal is probably what you want. Eggs can make the ideal brunch dish, or you can try something a bit more substantial such as Bulgar Kedgeree (page 86). If you find breakfast hard to face altogether, a nourishing drink or a plate of delicious fresh fruits could be the answer. The Strawberry Yogurt Drink on page 76 is full of vitamin C and would make the perfect refreshing start to a summer's morning.

Strawberry Yogurt Drink

This creamy breakfast drink, with its delicious blend of fruits, provides plenty of vitamin C, which is important for a healthy skin and the fight against infection.

SERVES 4
175 g (6 oz) strawberries, hulled
300 ml (½ pint) low-fat natural
yogurt
100 ml (4 fl oz) unsweetened
orange juice

5 ml (1 tsp) clear honey
2.5–5 ml (½–1 tsp) chopped
fresh mint
1 kiwi fruit, peeled and sliced
1 mandarin, peeled and
segmented

1 Slice four of the strawberries and put to one side. Coarsely chop the remainder, place in a blender or food processor with the yogurt, orange juice, honey and mint and purée until smooth.
2 Pour into four glasses and decorate with the strawberry, kiwi and mandarin slices. Serve with long spoons.

Nutritional analysis	
75 kcals/320 kJ	61 g Vitamin C ★ ★ ★ ★ ★
4.4 g Protein	159 mg Calcium ★ ★
0.9 g Fat	364 mg Potassium ★
13 g Carbohydrate	0.22 mg Riboflavin ★
1.4 g Fibre	

Fresh Fruit Platter

This makes an unusual and refreshing start to the day. The fruit and yogurt provide vitamin A in the form of carotene and retinol. Vitamin A deficiency leads to dry, scaly skin and dandruff.

SERVES 4
225 g (8 oz) fresh raspberries
150 ml (¼ pint) low-fat natural
yogurt
15 ml (1 tbsp) light muscovado
sugar
50 g (2 oz) redcurrants
4 ripe apricots, halved and
stoned

100 g (4 oz) white grapes
1 large pink grapefruit, peeled
and segmented
1 star fruit, sliced
1 small ripe mango, peeled,
stoned and sliced
90 ml (6 tbsp) unsweetened
apple juice
fresh mint leaves, to decorate

1 Purée the raspberries with the yogurt and sugar in a blender or food processor. Chill for 30 minutes. Sprinkle the prepared fruit with apple juice and leave to stand for 10 minutes.
2 Serve the prepared fruit, on a serving platter, decorated with mint leaves and accompanied by the raspberry and yogurt purée. Dip the fruit into the purée.

Nutritional analysis	
115 kcals/475 kJ	46.3 mg Vitamin C ★ ★ ★ ★ ★
3.4 g Protein	1.75 mcg Vitamin A ★ ★
0.5 g Fat	116 mg Calcium ★ ★
25.5 g Carbohydrate	1.5 mg Iron ★
7.1 g Fibre ★ ★	

Spiced Oatmeal Muffins

High-fibre muffins make a delicious treat for breakfast. These muffins provide some calcium – a mineral required, amongst other things, for maintaining substances which hold body cells together.

MAKES 12
175 g (6 oz) self raising wholemeal flour
50 g (2 oz) light muscovado sugar
50 g (2 oz) medium oatmeal
salt
5 ml (1 tsp) baking powder
2.5 ml (½ tsp) ground mixed spice
2.5 ml (½ tsp) ground cinnamon
1.25 ml (¼ tsp) freshly grated nutmeg
50 g (2 oz) raisins, rinsed
1 egg
300 ml (½ pint) semi-skimmed milk

1 Lightly grease 12 patty tins and set aside. Put all the dry in ingredients in a large bowl and mix well. Add the egg and milk and stir lightly until just mixed. Do not overbeat; the mixture should still be slightly lumpy.
2 Spoon the mixture into the prepared tins and bake at 200°C (400°F) mark 6 for 20–25 minutes or until well risen.

3 Turn out on to a wire rack and either serve at once, split and spread with a little polyunsaturated margarine, or allow them to cool and then split and toast before serving.

Nutritional analysis Per Muffin	
110 kcals/460 kJ	2.1 g Fibre
4 g Protein	51 mg Calcium ★
1.6 g Fat	1.1 mg Iron
21 g Carbohydrate	155 mg Potassium

Fruit Compote

This healthy fruit breakfast provides a good supply of vitamin B$_6$. B$_6$ is concerned with the metabolism of magnesium, zinc and essential fatty acids – all of which play an important part in the fight against inflammatory diseases and skin disorders.

SERVES 6
225 g (8 oz) dried whole bananas, chopped
225 g (8 oz) no-soak dried apricots, rinsed and quartered
grated rind and juice of 1 orange
grated rind and juice of 1 lemon
300 ml (½ pint) unsweetened orange juice
low-fat natural yogurt, to serve

1 Mix together the bananas, apricots, rinds and juice in a bowl. Pour over the orange juice and mix.
2 Cover and set aside to stand for at least 12 hours, stirring several times. Chill until ready to serve.

Nutritional analysis	
270 kcals/1124 kJ	54 mg Vitamin C ★ ★ ★ ★ ★
4.6 g Protein	305 mcg Vitamin A ★ ★ ★
0.7 g Fat	1.2 mg Vitamin B$_6$ ★ ★ ★
65 g Carbohydrate	1604 mg Potassium ★ ★ ★
17 g Fibre ★ ★ ★	

Mixed Nut and Seed Muesli

This muesli is an excellent source of iron, a mineral important to red blood cells which transport oxygen to all body cells, including those forming new skin.

SERVES 10

50 g (2 oz) shelled peanuts, with skins

50 g (2 oz) unsalted cashew nut pieces

25 g (1 oz) sunflower seeds

50 g (2 oz) pumpkin seeds

175 g (6 oz) barley flakes

175 g (6 oz) jumbo oats

1 Mix together the nuts and seeds and spread on a large baking sheet. Toast under a moderate grill, turning the ingredients occasionally, until lightly browned. Leave to cool.

2 Mix all the ingredients together and store in an airtight container.

3 Serve with semi-skimmed milk or low-fat natural yogurt and chopped fresh fruit.

Nutritional analysis	
220 kcals/925 kJ	8.7 mg Iron ★ ★ ★ ★
7.9 g Protein	0.35 mg Vitamin B$_1$ ★ ★
9.5 g Fat	4.1 mg Niacin ★ ★
28 g Carbohydrate	6.1 mg Vitamin C ★ ★
4.5 g Fibre ★	

Lemon Griddle Cakes With Strawberry Sauce

Strawberries provide both vitamin C and iron. The iron found in plant foods cannot be absorbed into the bloodstream unless vitamin C is also present.

MAKES 16

350 g (12 oz) strawberries, hulled and thawed if frozen

15 ml (1 tbsp) honey or light muscovado sugar

juice of ½ orange

50 g (2 oz) self raising flour

50 g (2 oz) self raising wholemeal flour

pinch of salt

1 egg

150 ml (¼ pint) semi-skimmed milk

finely grated rind of 1 lemon

1 Reserve a few whole strawberries for decoration, then gently cook the remainder with the honey or sugar and the orange juice in a covered saucepan for 5 minutes or until soft, stirring occasionally.

2 Remove the fruit from the saucepan, place in a bowl and leave to cool. Put the flours and salt into a bowl. Make a well in the centre and add the egg, milk and lemon rind. Beat together to form a smooth batter.

3 Spoon tablespoons of the batter on to a preheated non-stick griddle, allowing room for spreading. You will only be able to cook five or six at a time. Once the pancakes look puffy and bubbles appear on the surface, flip them over and cook until golden on the underside.

4 When cooked, wrap in a clean tea towel to keep warm while you cook the remaining batter. Serve warm with the reserved strawberries and cold fruit sauce.

Nutritional analysis Per Cake	
40 kcals/165 kJ	14 mg Vitamin C ★ ★ ★
1.6 g Protein	31 mg Calcium
0.7 g Fat	0.4 mg Iron
7.2 g Carbohydrate	74 mg Potassium
0.9 g Fibre	

Nut Soda Bread

This bread provides valuable amounts of potassium, calcium, iron and zinc. Zinc is one of the minerals often found to be deficient in our diet. A good intake is important to prevent acne and stretch marks.

MAKES 8 SLICES
350 g (12 oz) plain wholemeal flour
100 g (4 oz) plain flour
100 g (4 oz) walnut halves, chopped
2.5 ml (½ tsp) salt
5 ml (1 tsp) light muscovado sugar

5 ml (1 tsp) bicarbonate of soda
15 g (½ oz) polyunsaturated margarine
10 ml (2 tsp) cream of tartar
300 ml (½ pint) semi-skimmed milk
extra milk, to glaze

1 Lightly flour a baking sheet. Mix together the flours, walnuts (reserving some for decoration), salt, sugar and bicarbonate of soda, then rub in the margarine.

2 Dissolve the cream of tartar in the milk. Mix with the dry ingredients to make a soft dough, adding extra milk if necessary.

3 Knead on a lightly floured surface to a smooth dough. Shape into an 18 cm (7 inch) round and place on the baking sheet. Mark the top in a cross and brush with milk to glaze. Sprinkle with the reserved walnuts.

4 Bake at 200°C (400°F) mark 6 for about 40 minutes or until the bread is brown and sounds hollow when tapped on the bottom. Cool on a wire rack.

Nutritional analysis Per Slice	
285 kcals/1185 kJ	0.29 mg Vitamin B_1 ★ ★
9.7 g Protein	2.4 mg Iron ★ ★
9.7 g Fat	90 mg Calcium ★
42 g Carbohydrate	1.9 mg Zinc ★
5.3 g Fibre ★	

Devilled Poached Eggs

Minerals such as iron, calcium, potassium and zinc are present in this dish, together with a wide range of B complex vitamins, vitamins A, C, D and E. One serving provides nearly half the recommended daily amount (RDA) of vitamin E.

SERVES 4
15 ml (1 tbsp) polyunsaturated oil
1 small onion, skinned and finely chopped
6 tomatoes, seeded and chopped
100 g (4 oz) button mushrooms, chopped
5 ml (1 tsp) whole grain mustard
15 ml (1 tbsp) tomato purée
15 ml (1 tbsp) Worcestershire sauce
200 ml (7 fl oz) chicken stock
a few drops of Tabasco sauce
salt and pepper
5 ml (1 tsp) vinegar
4 eggs
4 slices of wholemeal bread

1 Heat the oil in a non-stick saucepan and fry the onion for 5 minutes or until softened. Add the tomatoes and mushrooms and simmer for a further 3 minutes.

2 Stir in the mustard, tomato purée, Worcestershire sauce, stock, Tabasco sauce and salt and pepper to taste. Simmer gently for 8 minutes.

3 If a smooth sauce is desired, put the sauce in a blender or food processor and blend for a few seconds. Keep hot.

4 Add the vinegar to a large frying pan of rapidly boiling water. Crack the eggs very carefully one at a time into a cup, then slide the eggs into the pan. Poach gently until the whites of the eggs are just set and the yolks are still runny.

5 Meanwhile, toast the bread. Place an egg on each slice of toast. Spoon the hot sauce over and serve immediately.

Nutritional analysis	
250 kcals/1045 kJ	31 mg Vitamin C ★ ★ ★ ★ ★
14 g Protein	4.6 mcg Vitamin E ★ ★ ★
12 g Fat	219 mcg Vitamin A ★ ★
23 g Carbohydrate	4 mg Iron ★ ★
6 g Fibre ★	

Brown Rice With Kidney and Bacon

Kidneys should be only just cooked or they will quickly toughen. Test frequently as their size will affect the cooking time. Kidneys are high in the B complex vitamins, vitamin E and minerals such as iron, copper and zinc. It is often difficult to ensure a good zinc intake, a mineral which is involved in many enzyme systems within the body.

SERVES 4
175 g (6 oz) long grain brown
rice
salt and pepper
100 g (4 oz) lean back bacon
450 g (1 lb) medium lamb's
kidneys
30 ml (2 tbsp) polyunsaturated
oil

15 g (½ oz) polyunsaturated
margarine
15 ml (1 tbsp) whole grain
mustard
200 ml (7 fl oz) unsweetened
apple juice
1 large eating apple

1 Cook the rice in plenty of boiling salted water for 30 minutes or until just tender. Drain, rinse and cool. Snip the bacon into large bite-sized pieces. Halve, skin and core the kidneys.
2 Heat the oil and margarine in a large frying pan. Add the bacon and cook until golden, stirring frequently. Remove from the pan. Add the kidneys and brown well.
3 Stir in the mustard followed by the rice and stir over a high heat for 1–2 minutes. Mix in the bacon and apple juice and season to taste with salt and pepper. Cover and simmer for about 6 minutes or until the kidneys are almost tender.
4 Meanwhile, quarter, core and roughly chop the apple. Stir into the kidneys, re-cover, and cook for 2–3 minutes. Adjust the seasoning before serving.

Nutritional analysis	
450 kcals/1880 kJ	1 mg Vitamin B_1 ★ ★ ★ ★ ★
29 g Protein	9.8 mg Iron ★ ★ ★ ★ ★
18 g Fat	4.5 mg Zinc ★ ★
47 g Carbohydrate	0.92 mg Copper ★ ★
2.5 g Fibre	

Devilled Kidneys

Serve these piquant kidneys with hot wholemeal toast. They contain all the essential nutrients for healthy red blood cells: vitamin B_{12}, folic acid and plenty of iron (three quarters of the recommended daily amount is provided in one portion).

SERVES 4
15 ml (1 tbsp) Worcestershire
sauce
15 ml (1 tbsp) tomato purée
10 ml (2 tsp) mustard powder
1.25 ml (¼ tsp) cayenne
15 g (½ oz) polyunsaturated
margarine

15 ml (1 tbsp) polyunsaturated
oil
8 lambs' kidneys, skinned,
halved and cored
parsley sprigs, to garnish

1 Whisk together the Worcestershire sauce, tomato purée, mustard powder, cayenne and margarine. Set aside.
2 Heat the oil in a large frying pan and cook the kidneys over a low heat for 3–4 minutes on each side or until they change colour.
3 Add the sauce mixture and cook for 2–3 minutes, stirring, until heated through. Garnish with parsley sprigs and serve at once.

Nutritional analysis	
180 kcals/750 kJ	9.1 mg Iron ★ ★ ★
20 g Protein	2 mg Vitamin B$_2$ ★ ★ ★ ★ ★
11 g Fat	62 mg Vitamin B$_{12}$ ★ ★ ★ ★ ★
1.3 g Carbohydrate	14 mg Vitamin C ★ ★ ★
0.1 g Fibre	40 mg Folic Acid ★

Scrambled Eggs with Tomato

This quick and easy breakfast dish provides the fat-soluble vitamins D and E. Vitamin E is important for the regeneration of new skin (for example at the site of a wound). Worcestershire sauce eliminates the need for extra salt.

SERVES 4
6 eggs, beaten
150 ml (¼ pint) semi-skimmed milk
15 g (½ oz) polyunsaturated margarine

2 tomatoes, coarsely chopped
dash of Worcestershire sauce
wholemeal toast, to serve

1 Beat together the eggs and milk. Melt the margarine in a non-stick saucepan over a low heat. Add the eggs and cook, stirring occasionally, until the eggs begin to scramble.
2 Add the tomatoes and Worcestershire sauce and continue cooking until set but still creamy. Serve at once with toast.

Nutritional analysis	
175 kcals/725 kJ	8.1 mg Vitamin C ★ ★
12 g Protein	2.7 mcg Vitamin E ★ ★
13 g Fat	0.48 mg Vitamin B_2 ★ ★
2.9 g Carbohydrate	2 mcg Vitamin D ★ ★
0.6 g Fibre	

Mushroom and Cashew Toasts

Coriander and parsley are rich in carotene, the precursor of vitamin A in the body. Apart from ensuring good low-light vision, vitamin A maintains healthy mucous membranes which help to prevent infection.

SERVES 4
450 g (1 lb) large flat or cup mushrooms
4 slices of wholemeal bread
45 ml (3 tbsp) polyunsaturated oil
15 g (½ oz) polyunsaturated margarine
50 g (2 oz) unsalted cashew nut pieces
75 ml (5 tbsp) chopped fresh coriander or parsley
15–30 ml (1–2) tbsp) lemon juice
salt and pepper
coriander or parsley sprigs, to garnish

1 Divide each mushroom into large wedge-shaped pieces. Toast the bread and keep warm.
2 Heat the oil and margarine in a large non-stick saucepan. Add the nuts and lightly brown, stirring frequently.
3 Add the mushrooms, cover and cook over a high heat for a few minutes only, shaking frequently. Mix in the coriander or parsley along with the lemon juice and salt and pepper to taste.
4 Spoon the mushrooms on to the slices of toast, along with all the pan juices, and serve immediately. Garnish with coriander or parsley sprigs.

Nutritional analysis	
305 kcals/1280 kJ	35 mg Vitamin C ★ ★ ★ ★ ★
8.8 g Protein	7.6 mcg Vitamin E ★ ★ ★ ★
22 g Fat	0.29 mg Vitamin B₁ ★ ★
19 g Carbohydrate	0.57 mg Vitamin B₂ ★ ★
8.1 g Fibre ★ ★	

Bulgar Kedgeree

This dish is high in vitamin B_{12} which is only found in foods of animal origin. It is vital for the formation of red blood cells. Other B complex vitamins are to be found in non-animal products as well.

SERVES 4
175 g (6 oz) bulgar wheat
2 kippers, about 450 g (1 lb)
total weight, heads and tails
removed
15 ml (1 tbsp) polyunsaturated
oil
1 small onion, chopped
pinch of cayenne

pepper
15 ml (1 tbsp) lemon juice
30 ml (2 tbsp) low-fat natural
yogurt
1 egg, hard-boiled and shelled,
white finely chopped and yolk
sieved
15 ml (1 tbsp) finely chopped
fresh parsley, to garnish

1 Put the bulgar wheat in a large bowl. Pour over 500 ml (17 fl oz) boiling water, stir and leave to soak for about 15 minutes.
2 Meanwhile, cook the kippers, covered, in 60 ml (4 tbsp) boiling water for 3 minutes. Remove from the heat and leave to stand for 5 minutes.
3 Drain the fish, reserving the liquor. Remove and discard all skin and bones and coarsely flake the fish.
4 Heat the oil in a non-stick saucepan and gently fry the onion for 3–5 minutes or until softened. Drain the bulgar wheat and add to the pan with the cayenne and pepper. Reduce the heat and cook very gently, for 5 minutes, stirring occasionally, until hot. Add the flaked fish, cover and leave to stand for 10 minutes.
5 Mix the lemon juice with 30 ml (2 tbsp) of the reserved fish liquor and the yogurt. Stir into the fish mixture with the chopped egg

white. Turn the kedgeree into a warmed serving dish and serve sprinkled with the egg yolk and the chopped parsley.

Nutritional analysis	
315 kcals/1315 kJ	5.7 mg Vitamin B$_{12}$ ★ ★ ★ ★
20 g Protein	0.46 mg Vitamin B$_6$ ★ ★
12 g Fat	3.9 mg Niacin ★ ★
35 g Carbohydrate	0.16 mg Vitamin B$_1$ ★
1.2 g Fibre	

2
Soups

Serve a nutritious home-made soup as an appetizer before a main course or as a meal in itself. You will find a wide range of soups to choose from in this chapter, from a warming Winter Vegetable Soup (overleaf), packed full of the goodness of fresh vegetables, to a chilled Red Cherry Soup (page 95) which can be served as an appetizer or a dessert. No matter whether a hearty or light soup, if you use fresh wholesome ingredients, it will add valuable nutrients to your diet.

Winter Vegetable Soup

This is a really substantial soup, best served as a meal in itself, with crusty granary bread or crisp bread rolls. It provides plenty of vitamin C which is important for a healthy skin. It is also high in fibre, important for a healthy digestive system.

SERVES 4
10 ml (2 tsp) lemon juice
225 g (8 oz) Jerusalem artichokes
½ small cabbage
450 g (1 lb) carrots
225 g (8 oz) turnips
2 onions, skinned, or 2 leeks, trimmed and washed
2–3 celery sticks, trimmed
1 bacon rasher, rinded and chopped

45 ml (3 tbsp) polyunsaturated oil
100 g (4 oz) haricot beans, soaked in cold water overnight and drained
bouquet garni
brown stock or water
salt and pepper
chopped fresh parsley and grated cheese, to serve

1 Fill a bowl with cold water and add the lemon juice. Peel the artichokes, slice them and then cut them into strips. Drop them into the acidulated water as you work, to prevent them from discolouring.
2 Shred the cabbage coarsely, discarding all thick or woody stalks. Cut the remaining vegetables into fairly small pieces.
3 In a large saucepan, fry the bacon lightly in its own fat. Add the oil and heat gently, then add all the vegetables (except the cabbage and beans) and fry for about 10 minutes, stirring, until soft but not coloured. Add the beans, bouquet garni and enough stock or water to cover. Add plenty of pepper and bring to the boil, then lower the heat, cover with a lid and simmer for 45 minutes–1 hour.
4 Add the cabbage and salt to taste. Cook for a further 20–30 minutes, adding more liquid as required. When all the ingredients are soft, discard the bouquet garni, taste and adjust the seasoning.

Serve the soup hot, sprinkled with chopped parsley, and with grated cheese handed separately.

Nutritional analysis	
260 kcals/1085 kJ	644 mcg Vitamin A ★ ★ ★ ★ ★
12 g Protein	74 mg Vitamin C ★ ★ ★ ★
12 g Fat	1280 mg Potassium ★ ★ ★
27 g Carbohydrate	243 mg Calcium ★ ★ ★
15 g Fibre ★ ★ ★	

Lettuce And Mange-Tout Soup

This soup provides plenty of carotene (or vitamin A), as well as vitamin C. Both vitamins play an important role in the body's defence system.

SERVES 4
15 ml (1 tbsp) polyunsaturated oil
2 shallots, skinned and chopped
30 ml (2 tbsp) chopped celery leaves
900 ml (1½ pints) chicken or vegetable stock, skimmed
225 g (8 oz) mange-tout

½ cos lettuce
5 ml (1 tsp) reduced-sodium soy sauce, preferably naturally fermented shoyu
pepper
15 ml (1 tbsp) chopped fresh mint or lemon balm
45 ml (3 tbsp) chopped fresh parsley or chervil

1 Heat the oil in a large saucepan. Add the shallots and fry gently for about 5 minutes or until softened. Add the celery leaves and stock and bring to the boil. Simmer, partly covered, for 5 minutes.
2 Meanwhile, string the mange-tout and cut in half if large. Finely shred the lettuce. Add these to the pan with the soy sauce and pepper to taste, then bring back to the boil.
3 Simmer for 5 minutes or until the lettuce is wilted, then stir in the herbs. Serve hot.

Nutritional analysis	
80 kcals/335 kJ	209 mcg Vitamin A ★ ★
4.6 g Protein	37 mg Vitamin C ★ ★ ★ ★ ★
4.1 g Fat	2.2 mcg Vitamin E ★ ★
6.9 g Carbohydrate	2.6 mg Iron ★ ★
4.7 g Fibre ★	

Spinach Soup

Spinach is a source of folic acid, a B vitamin involved in protein production. Proteins are required for cells, hormones and enzymes, and are constantly being renewed. Folic acid is a very important vitamin for pregnant women.

SERVES 4
450 g (1 lb) fresh spinach
900 ml (1½ pints) vegetable or chicken stock, skimmed

15 ml (1 tbsp) lemon juice
salt and pepper
450 ml (¾ pint) buttermilk
a few drops of Tabasco sauce

1 Strip the spinach leaves from their stems and wash in several changes of water. Place the spinach, stock and lemon juice in a large saucepan and add salt and pepper to taste. Bring to the boil, then simmer for 10 minutes.

2 Work the spinach through a sieve, or strain off most of the liquid and reserve, then purée the spinach in a blender or food processor.

3 Reheat the spinach purée gently with the cooking liquid, 300 ml (½ pint) of the buttermilk and the Tabasco sauce. Swirl in the remaining buttermilk just before serving.

Nutritional analysis	
80 kcals/335 kJ	1055 mcg Vitamin A ★ ★ ★ ★ ★
7 g Protein	34 mg Vitamin C ★ ★ ★ ★ ★
1.9 g Fat	13 mg Iron ★ ★ ★ ★ ★
9.5 g Carbohydrate	144 mg Folic Acid ★ ★ ★
0.7 g Fibre	

Watercress Soup

Watercress, like other dark green leafy vegetables, is a good source of calcium. Milk and milk products are the other main sources of calcium, vital for strong bones and teeth. Try serving this delicately flavoured soup with a swirl of Greek strained yogurt over the top of each portion.

SERVES 4
15 g (½ oz) polyunsaturated margarine
1 small onion, skinned and chopped
1 bunch of watercress, trimmed and coarsely chopped
20 g (¾ oz) plain wholemeal flour
300 ml (½ pint) chicken or vegetable stock, skimmed
300 ml (½ pint) semi-skimmed milk
1.25 ml (¼ tsp) freshly grated nutmeg
salt and pepper
watercress sprigs and paprika, to garnish

1 Melt the margarine in a saucepan. Add the onion and watercress and cook over a low heat for 3–5 minutes or until the onion is soft but not brown, stirring occasionally.

2 Add the flour and cook for 1 minute, then gradually stir in the stock, milk and nutmeg. Bring to the boil, stirring. Add salt and

pepper to taste, lower the heat and simmer, covered, for about 15 minutes or until thickened and smooth.

3 Remove from the heat and leave to cool slightly, then purée in a blender or food processor. Return the soup to the saucepan and reheat. Serve in individuals bowls garnished with watercress sprigs and a sprinkling of paprika.

Nutritional analysis	
90 kcals/370 kJ	133 mg Calcium ★ ★
4.1 g Protein	11 mg Vitamin C ★ ★
4.6 Fat	1.1 mcg Vitamin E ★
8.3 g Carbohydrate	41 mg Folic Acid ★
1.1 g Fibre	

Cold Cucumber Soup

Calcium, phosphorus, potassium, zinc and iron are the minerals present in useful amounts in this cool, creamy and refreshing soup. Potassium acts as an essential activator in a number of enzymes, particularly those concerned with energy production.

SERVES 4
2 medium cucumbers, peeled
100 g (4 oz) walnuts, chopped
30 ml (2 tbsp) olive oil or a mixture of walnut and olive oil
300 ml (½ pint) chicken stock, skimmed
1 garlic clove, skinned and crushed
30 ml (2 tbsp) chopped fresh dill or
10 ml (2 tsp) dried dill
salt and pepper
300 ml (½ pint) low-fat natural yogurt
sprigs of fresh dill, to garnish

1 Cut the cucumbers into small dice and place in a bowl. Add the walnuts, oil, stock, garlic and chopped or dried dill and season to taste with salt and pepper.

2 Stir the soup well, cover the bowl and chill in the refrigerator for at least 8 hours, or overnight.

3 To serve, uncover and whisk in the yogurt. Ladle into chilled individual soup bowls surrounded by crushed ice, and garnish with sprigs of dill.

Nutritional analysis	
265 kcals/1105 kJ	18 mg Vitamin C ★ ★ ★
8.1 g Protein	204 mg Calcium ★ ★ ★
21 g Fat .	678 mg Potassium ★ ★
11 g Carbohydrate	1.4 mg Zinc ★
2.2 g Fibre	

Avocado Soup

This chilled avocado soup has a delicate lemony flavour. Avocados are a valuable source of vitamin E – the vitamin responsible for protecting essential fatty acids in the body. This vitamin also pro-tects vitamins A and C, both of which are also found in avocados.

SERVES 4
1 large, ripe avocado
450 ml (¾ pint) chicken stock,
skimmed
30 ml (2 tbsp) lemon juice

200 ml (7 fl oz) milk
5 ml (1 tsp) honey
pinch of cayenne
salt and pepper
2 ripe tomatoes, to garnish

1 Halve the avocado, discard the stone and peel and roughly chop the flesh.
2 Put the avocado in a blender or food processor with the chicken stock, lemon juice, milk, honey and cayenne and blend until smooth. Season to taste with salt and pepper. Pour into a bowl, cover and chill in the refrigerator for no longer than 2 hours. (The soup will begin to discolour if you leave it any longer).
3 Meanwhile, blanch the tomatoes in boiling water for 10 seconds, then peel. Halve the tomatoes, remove the seeds, then cut each half into thin slivers.
4 Taste and adjust the seasoning of the soup. Garnish with the tomato slivers just before serving.

Nutritional analysis	
230 kcals/970 kJ	62 mg Vitamin C ★ ★ ★ ★ ★
6.4 g Protein	3.2 mcg Vitamin E ★ ★
20 g Fat	0.46 mg Vitamin B_6 ★ ★
7.6 g Carbohydrate	649 mg Potassium ★ ★
2.3 g Fibre	

Red Cherry Soup

There is enough potassium in a portion of this soup to maintain a normal water balance within body cells and prevent fluid retention.

SERVES 4
450 g (1 lb) fresh red cherries
15 ml (1 tbsp) light muscovado sugar
150 ml (¼ pint) red wine

1 cinnamon stick
pared rind of ½ lemon
150 ml (¼ pint) low-fat natural yogurt or smetana

1 Stone the cherries and reserve the stones. Reserve a few cherries for garnish. Put the remainder into a stainless steel or enamel saucepan with 150 ml (¼ pint) water and the sugar. Bring to the boil and simmer gently for 10 minutes or until completely soft.
2 Wrap half the cherry stones loosely in a clean tea towel and, using a heavy rolling pin, crack the stones to reveal the kernels.
3 Put the cracked stones in a clean saucepan with the reserved whole cherry stones, the wine, cinnamon stick and lemon rind. Bring to the boil and simmer for 5–10 minutes, then strain the liquid into the cherry mixture.
4 Sieve or purée the soup in a blender or food processor, then leave to cool for 30 minutes.
5 Stir the yogurt or smetana into the cherry pulp and chill in the refrigerator for at least 2 hours. Garnish with the reserved cherries before serving.

Nutritional analysis	
115 kcals/470 kJ	457 mg Potassium ★
2.6 g Protein	90 mg Calcium ★
0.4 g Fat	0.18 mg Vitamin B_2 ★
20 g Carbohydrate	5.8 mg Vitamin C ★
1.9 g Fibre	

Gazpacho

One portion of this traditional chilled Spanish soup provides 86 mg of vitamin C which is nearly three times the recommended daily amount. Vitamin C plays many roles within the body and a deficiency of it can lead to scurvy and the breakdown of skin at the site of old wounds.

SERVES 4

225 g (8 oz) tomatoes, seeded and finely diced
⅓ cucumber, peeled, seeded and finely diced
1 onion, skinned and chopped
1 small green pepper, cored, seeded and diced
1 small red pepper, cored, seeded and diced
1 garlic clove, skinned and finely chopped
450 ml (¾ pint) tomato juice, chilled

150 ml (¼ pint) chicken or vegetable stock, skimmed and chilled
15 ml (1 tbsp) olive oil
45 ml (3 tbsp) red wine vinegar
a few drops of Tabasco sauce
salt and pepper
a few sprigs of fresh chervil, to garnish
TO SERVE
2 slices of wholemeal bread, toasted and cubed
ice cubes

1 Reserve about a quarter of the tomatoes, cucumber, onion and peppers for the garnish. Place the remaining vegetables in a blender or food processor with the garlic and tomato juice and blend until smooth.

2 Add the stock, oil, vinegar and Tabasco sauce and blend well. Add salt and pepper to taste. Pour into a bowl, cover and chill for about 30 minutes.

3 Stir the soup and garnish with the chervil. Serve with the reserved vegetables, wholemeal bread croûtons and ice cubes in separate bowls, to be added to the soup as desired.

Nutritional analysis	
80 kcals/335 kJ	86 mg Vitamin C ★ ★ ★ ★ ★
2.4 g Protein	166 mcg Vitamin A ★ ★
4 g Fat	658 mg Potassium ★ ★
9 g Carbohydrate	1.4 mg Iron ★
2 g Fibre	

Sweetcorn and Haddock Chowder

This is a low-fat soup: cod and haddock are both low-fat fish and using semi-skimmed milk reduces the fat content further. Vitamins B_2 and B_{12} are present in important quantities.

SERVES 4
15 g (½ oz) polyunsaturated margarine
1 onion, skinned and finely chopped
225 g (8 oz) naturally smoked haddock fillet
225 g (8 oz) cod fillet
1 bay leaf
1 thin strip of lemon rind

450 ml (¾ pint) semi-skimmed milk
300 ml (½ pint) dry white wine
pepper
90 ml (6 tbsp) drained canned sweetcorn
30 ml (2 tbsp) chopped fresh parsley
1 egg, hard-boiled and finely chopped, to garnish

1 Melt the margarine in a large non-stick saucepan and cook the onion gently for 3 minutes.
2 Add the fish, bay leaf, lemon rind, milk, wine and pepper to taste. Bring to the boil, then lower the heat and simmer, covered, for 15 minutes.
3 Using a slotted spoon, remove about 60 ml (4 tbsp) fish and set aside. Remove the bay leaf and lemon rind and discard.
4 Put the soup in a blender or food processor and purée until smooth.
5 Return the soup to the rinsed-out saucepan, add the sweetcorn, reserved fish and parsley and heat gently until piping hot.
6 Serve in soup bowls, with chopped hard-boiled egg sprinkled on top.

Nutritional analysis	
265 kcals/1105 kJ	207 mg Calcium ★ ★ ★
27 g Protein	2.8 mg Vitamin B₁₂ ★ ★ ★ ★ ★
7.5 g Fat	16 mg Vitamin C ★ ★ ★
11 g Carbohydrate	0.42 mg Vitamin B₂ ★ ★
2.2 g Fibre	

3
Starters

The ideal starter should look appealing, stimulate the appetite and complement the food to follow. This chapter contains an inspiring selection of attractive and appetizing starters ranging from a simple fruit cocktail (page 107) and a crunchy raw vegetable salad (page 100) to Crab-stuffed Avocado (page 103) and Asparagus with Orange Sauce (page 100) for a special occasion. It is important that a starter should look attractive, especially when entertaining, as it is the first thing your guests will see. Use garnishes, such as decoratively cut fresh fruit and vegetables, or a sprinkling of chopped fresh herbs, to add colour and interest to the dishes.

Grated Raw Vegetables with Garlic Dressing

Packed with carotene (vitamin A), one portion of this crunchy vegetable mix provides more than the recommended daily amount of this vitamin. Deficiency in vitamin A can lead to dry, scaly skin and dandruff.

SERVES 4
175 g (6 oz) carrots
175 g (6 oz) courgettes, trimmed
175 g (6 oz) celeriac
15 ml (1 tbsp) lemon juice
175 g (6 oz) raw beetroot
90 ml (6 tbsp) olive oil
30 ml (2 tbsp) wine vinegar

2.5 ml (½ tsp) light muscovado sugar
2.5 ml (½ tsp) mustard powder
1 large garlic clove, skinned and crushed
salt and pepper
chopped fresh parsley, to garnish

1 Grate the carrots, avoiding the central core. Grate the courgettes and mix with the carrots in a salad bowl.
2 Peel and grate the celeriac, toss immediately in the lemon juice and add to the carrot and courgette mixture. Lastly, peel and grate the beetroot and add to the mixture.
3 Put the oil, vinegar, sugar, mustard and garlic in a screw-topped jar with salt and pepper to taste. Shake the jar until the dressing is well blended.
4 Pour the dressing over the vegetables and toss lightly just to coat. Serve immediately, garnished with chopped parsley.

Nutritional analysis	
245 kcals/1030 kJ	905 mcg Vitamin A ★ ★ ★ ★ ★
2.5 g Protein	15 mg Vitamin C ★ ★ ★
23 g Fat	549 mg Potassium ★
8.6 g Carbohydrate	1.2 mg Iron ★
5.1 g Fibre ★	

Asparagus with Orange Sauce

Make the most of the fresh asparagus season and serve this luxurious but healthy starter. It contains a range of vitamins and minerals, including vitamins C and E and potassium.

SERVES 4
450 g (1 lb) fresh asparagus, trimmed and scraped
150 ml (¼ pint) dry white wine
juice of 1 orange

150 ml (¼ pint) Greek-style natural yogurt
1 egg, size 2
salt

TO GARNISH   *orange slices*
finely pared rind of 1 orange,
finely shredded

1 Tie the asparagus in a bundle and cover the tips with a cap of foil. Stand, tips uppermost, in a deep saucepan of boiling water, lower the heat and simmer for 15 minutes or until tender. Drain and arrange in a serving dish.
2 Meanwhile, place the wine and orange juice in a small saucepan and boil for 7–8 minutes or until reduced by two-thirds.
3 Beat together the yogurt and egg in a small heatproof bowl over a pan of simmering water. Cook for about 10 minutes, whisking continuously until thickened, then gradually stir in the reduced liquid. Add salt to taste and spoon the sauce over the asparagus tips. Garnish with finely shredded orange rind and orange slices.

Nutritional analysis	
110 kcals/450 kJ	19 mg Vitamin C ★ ★ ★ ★
5 g Protein	0.83 mcg Vitamin E ★
5.3 g Fat	210 mg Potassium
4.5 g Carbohydrate	70 mg Calcium
0.6 g Fibre	

Basil and Tomato Tartlets

Make these tarts in the summer when fresh basil is available. Don't be tempted to use dried basil instead as the flavour is quite different. These tartlets are particularly high in calcium – an important mineral which, amongst other things, helps to control the 'excitability' of nerves and muscles.

SERVES 4   *6 tomatoes, roughly chopped*
75 g (3 oz) plain wholemeal flour *200 g (7 oz) Mozzarella cheese,*
75 g (3 oz) plain white flour   *cut into 1 cm (½ inch) cubes*
50 g (2 oz) polyunsaturated   *45 ml (3 tbsp) chopped fresh*
margarine   *basil*
50 g (2 oz) Cheddar cheese,   *salt and pepper*
grated   *basil leaves, to garnish*
1 egg yolk

1 To make the pastry, put the flours in a bowl and rub in the margarine until the mixture resembles fine breadcrumbs.

2 Stir in the Cheddar cheese and the egg yolk mixed with 30 ml (2 tbsp) water. Knead on a lightly floured surface to form a smooth, firm dough.
3 Divide the dough into four equal pieces and roll out each piece on a lightly floured surface. Use to line four 10 cm (4 inch) flan tins or dishes.
4 Bake blind at 200°C (400°F) mark 6 for 10 minutes. Remove the paper and beans and bake for a further 10 minutes. Cool, then remove from the tins.
5 Mix together the tomatoes, Mozzarella and chopped basil and season to taste with salt and pepper. Divide the filling between the pastry cases, garnish with basil and serve at once.

Nutritional analysis	
445 kcals/1865 kJ	416 mg Calcium ★ ★ ★ ★ ★
19 g Protein	2.8 mg Zinc ★ ★
28 g Fat	20 mg Vitamin C ★ ★ ★ ★
31 g Carbohydrate	5.3 mcg Vitamin E ★ ★ ★
3.9 g Fibre ★	

Shredded Spinach with Smoked Ham

Spinach is an excellent source of carotene (which the body transforms into vitamin A), vitamin C and vitamin E. Vitamin E protects both C and A from destruction within the body. To serve as a main course, increase the amount of ham and add a few lightly boiled potatoes.

SERVES 6
225 g (8 oz) fresh spinach
100 g (4 oz) sliced lean smoked ham
15 ml (1 tbsp) whole grain mustard

45 ml (3 tbsp) polyunsaturated oil
15 ml (1 tbsp) olive oil
15 ml (1 tbsp) lemon juice
salt and pepper
2 ripe pears

1 Pull any coarse stalks off the spinach. Wash the leaves well, drain, then shred roughly. Cut the ham into small pieces, mix with the spinach and place in a salad bowl.
2 Whisk together the mustard, oils, lemon juice and salt and pepper to taste. Peel, quarter, core and slice the pears into the

dressing. Stir well to mix, then toss with the spinach and ham. Serve immediately.

Nutritional analysis	
160 kcals/660 kJ	350 mcg Vitamin A ★ ★ ★
7.4 g Protein	13 mg Vitamin C ★ ★ ★
12 g Fat	4.5 mcg Vitamin E ★ ★ ★
6.1 g Carbohydrate	4.6 mg Iron ★ ★
1.2 g Fibre	

Crab-Stuffed Avocado

One serving of this starter provides valuable amounts of vitamin B₆, the vitamin which regulates the body's fluid balance by controlling potassium and sodium levels.

SERVES 4
2 ripe avocados
175 g (6 oz) fresh white crab meat or 175 g (6 oz) can crab meat, drained and flaked
2 spring onions, trimmed and finely chopped
30 ml (2 tbsp) lemon juice
45 ml (3 tbsp) olive oil
1 small garlic clove, skinned and crushed
5 ml (1 tsp) curry powder
pepper
45 ml (3 tbsp) fresh wholemeal breadcrumbs
15 ml (1 tbsp) grated Parmesan cheese

1 Cut the avocados in half, discard the stones and scoop out the flesh to within 3 mm (1/8 inch) of the skin. Place the avocado shells in a shallow ovenproof dish and set aside. Chop the avocado flesh into small cubes and place in a mixing bowl. Add the crab meat and spring onions.
2 Put the lemon juice, olive oil, garlic and curry powder in a screw-topped jar. Add pepper to taste and shake until well blended. Pour the dressing over the crab mixture and toss well.
3 Pile the mixture into the avocado shells. Mix the breadcrumbs and Parmesan cheese together and sprinkle over the top of the avocados.
4 Bake at 200°C (400°F) mark 6 for 10–15 minutes or until the topping is crisp. Serve immediately.

Nutritional analysis	
450 kcals/1875 kJ	22 mg Vitamin C ★ ★ ★ ★
15 g Protein	4.5 mcg Vitamin E ★ ★ ★
40 g Fat	0.53 mg Vitamin B$_6$ ★ ★
7.8 g Carbohydrate	3.1 mg Zinc ★ ★
3.5 g Fibre ★	

Kipper Mousse

When buying kippers, check for plump flesh and an oily skin – these are signs of quality. A dark-brown colour does not necessarily mean a good kipper, as this is probably an artificial dye. This mousse is rich in vitamins D and B$_{12}$, together with valuable amounts of vitamin B$_6$. Vitamin D, like vitamins A and C, also stimulates the healing of skin.

SERVES 4
350 g (12 oz) naturally smoked kipper fillets
juice of 1 orange
15 ml (1 tbsp) lemon juice
5 ml (1 tsp) gelatine
100 g (4 oz) plain fromage frais
150 ml (¼ pint) low-fat natural yogurt
1 small garlic clove, skinned and crushed
1.25 ml (¼ pint) ground mace
salt and pepper
lemon or orange slices and herb sprigs, to garnish

1 Pour boiling water over the kippers and leave to stand for 1 minute. Drain and remove the skin. Flake the flesh, discarding any large bones, and put in a blender or food processor.
2 In a small heatproof bowl, mix the orange and lemon juices together. Sprinkle on the gelatine and leave to stand for a few minutes or until spongy.
3 Meanwhile, add the fromage frais, yogurt, garlic and mace to the blender or food processor and blend with the kippers until smooth.
4 Place the bowl of gelatine in a saucepan of hot water and heat gently until dissolved. Add to the kipper mixture and blend until evenly mixed. Add salt and pepper to taste.
5 Divide the kipper mousse equally between four oiled ramekin dishes. Chill in the refrigerator for at least 1 hour before serving.

6 Turn the mousses out on to individual plates and garnish with lemon or orange slices and herb sprigs. Serve with wholemeal toast.

Nutritional analysis	
230 kcals/950 kJ	0.55 mg Vitamin B_6 ★ ★
29 g Protein	25 mg Vitamin C ★ ★ ★ ★ ★
10 g Fat	22 mcg Vitamin D ★ ★ ★ ★ ★
5.1 g Carbohydrate	9.8 mg Vitamin B_{12} ★ ★ ★ ★ ★
1.1 g Fibre	.

Smoked Chicken and Mint Salad

Smoked chickens can be found in delicatessens and some supermarkets. The moist, tasty flesh is rich and benefits from the freshness of mint, cucumber and strawberries. A good range of B complex vitamins is provided per serving of this salad; these are required by the body for energy production, as well as for maintaining healthy skin, blood, nervous and immune systems.

SERVES 6
1.1 kg (2½ lb) smoked chicken
1 small cucumber
100 g (4 oz) strawberries, hulled
150 g (5 oz) Greek-style natural yogurt
45 ml (3 tbsp) chopped fresh mint
salt and pepper
mint sprigs, to garnish

1 Thinly slice the chicken breast, leaving on the skin. Cut the leg flesh into strips, discarding the skin. Thinly slice half the cucumber and all the strawberries. Tightly cover all these ingredients and refrigerate.
2 Coarsely grate the remaining cucumber and mix into the yogurt with the chopped mint and salt and pepper to taste. Cover tightly and refrigerate.
3 About 30 minutes before serving, arrange some of the chicken, cucumber and strawberry slices on each of six individual serving plates. Pile the chicken leg flesh in the centre of each and top with a small spoonful of the yogurt dressing.
4 Garnish the salads with mint sprigs and serve the remaining dressing separately.

Nutritional analysis	
270 kcals/1135 kJ	9.3 mg Niacin ★ ★ ★
32 g Protein	0.12 mg Vitamin B_1 ★
15 g Fat	0.37 mg Vitamin B_6 ★
3.4 g Carbohydrate	18 mg Vitamin C ★ ★ ★
0.8 g Fibre ★ ★	2 mg Zinc ★

Warm Whitebait Salad

This salad is best served when still slightly warm. Whitebait is an oily fish which provides essential fatty acids, together with the omega-3 fatty acids thought to be beneficial to psoriasis sufferers. This salad is exceptionally high in vitamin E, the vitamin which protects these polyunsaturated fatty acids.

SERVES 4
100 g (4 oz) French beans
lettuce leaves
polyunsaturated oil
juice of 2 large limes

1.25 ml (¼ tsp) chilli powder
salt and pepper
225 g (8 oz) whitebait
flour

1 Top, tail and halve the French beans. Blanch in boiling salted water for 3 minutes, drain and cool. Rinse, drain and dry the lettuce leaves.
2 Whisk together 60 ml (4 tbsp) of the oil, the lime juice, chilli powder and salt and pepper to taste.
3 Rinse, drain and dry the whitebait. Toss in a little seasoned flour then deep fry in hot oil until golden brown. Drain on absorbent kitchen paper.
4 While still warm, toss the whitebait and beans together with the dressing. Cool slightly before serving on a bed of lettuce leaves.

Nutritional analysis	
435 kcals/1820 kJ	19 mcg Vitamin E ★ ★ ★ ★ ★
11 g Protein	12 mg Vitamin C ★ ★
42 g Fat	499 mg Calcium ★ ★ ★ ★
4 g Carbohydrate	3.2 mg Iron ★ ★
1.2 g Fibre	

Melon and Grape Cocktail

This light starter contains plenty of carotene (vitamin A) and vita-
min C. Raw fruit and vegetables play an important part in a healthy
diet and help keep skin in good condition.

SERVES 4
1 large Galia or Charentais
melon, halved and seeded
175 g (6 oz) black grapes, halved
and seeded
75 g (3 oz) seedless green grapes

juice of 2 oranges
juice of 2 limes
pinch of ground mixed spice
fresh mint sprigs, to garnish
(optional)

1 Scoop the melon flesh into balls with a melon baller, or peel and
cut into fine dice.
2 Mix the melon in a bowl with the grapes, orange juice, lime juice
and mixed spice. Cover and chill for 3–4 hours. Serve garnished
with sprigs of mint, if liked.

Nutritional analysis	
72 kcals/301 kJ	377 mcg Vitamin A ★ ★ ★
1.6 g Protein	49 mg Vitamin C ★ ★ ★ ★ ★
0 g Fat	579 mg Potassium ★
17 g Carbohydrate	1.2 mg Iron ★
1.4 g Fibre	

4

Light Meals and Snacks

The recipes in this chapter will be useful for family lunches and suppers and for children's teas, although some, such as Mussels in Tomato Sauce (page 114), could be reserved for an informal supper or lunch party. Many of them combine traditional foods with new ideas, such as Baked Jacket Potatoes with Hummus (page 121) and Goat's Cheese Tarts (page 120), to create new and deliciously nutritious combinations of flavours. With such a mouthwatering selection to choose from, there will be no need to rely on less healthy convenience foods for your light meals and snacks.

Warm Chicken Liver and Bread Salad

On cold days, warm salads make an interesting change from the traditional chilled variety. This one is rich in vitamins and minerals, iron, folic acid, and vitamin B_{12} being the most valuable because all are vital for red blood cell production and all can be deficient in some people's diets.

SERVES 4
400 g (14 oz) can chick-peas, rinsed and drained
1 large green pepper, cored, seeded and cut into thin strips
½ cucumber, chopped
100 g (4 oz) cherry tomatoes, halved
1 small onion, skinned and sliced
30 ml (2 tbsp) coarsely chopped fresh parsley
15 g (½ oz) polyunsaturated margarine

45 ml (3 tbsp) polyunsaturated oil
100 g (4 oz) button mushrooms, halved
225 g (8 oz) chicken livers, trimmed and chopped
2 slices of wholemeal bread
30 ml (2 tbsp) red wine
2 garlic cloves, skinned and crushed
salt and pepper

1 Put the chick-peas in a bowl with the other vegetables and parsley.
2 Heat the margarine and 15 ml (1 tbsp) oil in a frying pan and cook the mushrooms for 2 minutes, stirring all the time. Add the chicken livers and cook for about 4 minutes or until cooked through and evenly coloured but still slightly pink in the centre.
3 Meanwhile, lightly toast the bread. Chop roughly and add to the salad.
4 Using a slotted spoon, transfer the mushrooms and livers to the salad bowl. Quickly add the remaining oil, wine and garlic to the frying pan and heat until bubbling. Season to taste with salt and pepper. Pour over the salad, toss together and serve immediately.

Nutritional analysis	
340 kcals/1415 kJ	85 mg Vitamin C ★ ★ ★ ★ ★
18 g Protein	7.4 mcg Vitamin E ★ ★ ★ ★
22 g Fat	385 mg Folic Acid ★ ★ ★ ★ ★
19 g Carbohydrate	32 mg Vitamin B_{12} ★ ★ ★ ★ ★
7.4 g Fibre ★ ★	4.3 mg Iron ★ ★ ★

Prawn Risotto

Shellfish are a source of minerals, including copper which assists many enzymes, such as those needed for the production of melanin – the pigment which gives skin and hair their characteristic colour.

SERVES 4
1 small onion, skinned and thinly sliced
1 garlic clove, skinned and crushed
1 litre (1¾ pints) chicken stock, skimmed
225 g (8 oz) long grain brown rice
50 g (2 oz) small button mushrooms
½ sachet saffron threads
salt and pepper
225 g (8 oz) cooked peeled prawns
50 g (2 oz) frozen petits pois
12 whole cooked prawns, to garnish

1 Place the onion, garlic, stock, rice, mushrooms and saffron in a large saucepan or flameproof casserole. Add salt and pepper to taste. Bring to the boil and simmer, uncovered, for 35 minutes, stirring occasionally.
2 Stir in the prawns and petits pois. Cook over a high heat for about 5 minutes or until most of the liquid has been absorbed, stirring occasionally.
3 Taste and adjust the seasoning, then turn into a warmed serving dish. Garnish with the whole prawns and serve immediately.

Nutritional analysis	
290 kcals/1220 kJ	121 mg Calcium ★ ★
21 g Protein	2.5 mg Iron ★ ★
3 g Fat	1.1 mg Copper ★ ★
48 g Carbohydrate	0.39 mg Vitamin B$_1$ ★ ★
4.4 g Fibre ★	

Bean and Chicken Tabouleh

Tabouleh is a traditional Middle Eastern dish. It is made with bulgar wheat which is available at health food shops. This substantial salad is a variation on the classic recipe. The vitamin C encourages better absorption of the iron that is also present in the dish.

SERVES 4
150 g (5 oz) bulgar wheat
400 g (14 oz) can red kidney beans, drained and rinsed
4 spring onions, trimmed and finely chopped
1 garlic clove, skinned and crushed
60 ml (4 tbsp) chopped fresh mint

30 ml (2 tbsp) chopped fresh parsley
60 ml (4 tbsp) olive oil
juice of 1 lemon
salt and pepper
175 g (6 oz) cooked chicken meat, skinned and chopped
lettuce leaves and mint and parsley sprigs, to serve

1 Soak the bulgar wheat in cold water for 35–40 minutes or until soft. Drain off the excess liquid, pressing the bulgar to squeeze out the moisture. This can be done by putting the drained bulgar into a clean tea towel and lightly squeezing the towel.
2 Mix together the prepared bulgar wheat, the kidney beans, spring onions, garlic, mint and parsley.
3 Mix the oil with the lemon juice and salt and pepper to taste, then stir into the bulgar wheat and beans. Mix in the cooked chicken and leave for at least 30 minutes to let the flavours develop. Serve the tabouleh on a bed of lettuce leaves garnished with herb sprigs.

Nutritional analysis	
390 kcals/1625 kJ	17 mg Vitamin C ★ ★ ★
20 g Protein	0.28 mg Vitamin B$_1$ ★ ★
18 g Fat	4.3 mg Iron ★ ★
39 g Carbohydrate	622 mg Potassium ★ ★
6.5 g Fibre ★ ★	

Seafood Spaghetti

High in fibre, this dish also provides more than the recommended daily amount (RDA) of iron and vitamin B_1. Vitamin B_1, like vitamin C, is a particularly vulnerable vitamin liable to be destroyed during food preparation.

SERVES 4
450 g (1 lb) wholewheat spaghetti
1 small onion, skinned and chopped
300 ml (½ pint) dry white wine
2 egg yolks
100 g (4 oz) natural Quark

175 g (6 oz) cooked white fish, boned and flaked
100 g (4 oz) cooked fresh or canned shelled mussels
100 g (4 oz) cooked fresh or canned shelled cockles
salt and pepper

1 Cook the spaghetti in a large saucepan of fast-boiling lightly salted water for about 10 minutes or until tender.
2 Meanwhile, put the onion and white wine in a saucepan and simmer very gently for 3–4 minutes, without allowing the wine to evaporate too much. Remove from the heat and whisk in the egg yolks, one at a time, followed by the natural Quark. Add the white fish, mussels and cockles. Heat through gently and add salt and pepper to taste.
3 Drain the pasta and put in a serving dish. Spoon the sauce over the pasta and serve immediately.

Nutritional analysis	
555 kcals/2320 kJ	1 mg Vitamin B_1 ★ ★ ★ ★ ★
36 g Protein	2.3 mcg Vitamin E ★ ★
8.5 g Fat	16 g Iron ★ ★ ★ ★ ★
77 g Carbohydrate	5.1 mg Zinc ★ ★ ★
11 g Fibre ★ ★	

Mussels in Tomato Sauce

Mussels should always be bought alive; check by tapping any open shells with the handle of a knife and discard any that don't close immediately. Serve with lots of bread to mop up the delicious juices. Shellfish and crustaceans are concentrated sources of minerals such as iron and calcium.

SERVES 2
1.1 kg (2½ lb) or 2.8 litres (5 pints) fresh mussels
40 g (1½ oz) coarse oatmeal
450 g (1 lb) ripe tomatoes
15 ml (1 tbsp) polyunsaturated oil
1 small onion, skinned and finely chopped
1 garlic clove, skinned and crushed

5 ml (1 tsp) dried thyme
15 ml (1 tbsp) tomato purée
5 ml (1 tsp) white wine vinegar
300 ml (½ pint) dry cider
salt and pepper
chopped fresh parsley, to garnish

1 Pick over the mussels, discarding any that have open or damaged shells. Scrub the shells under cold running water to remove any sand or grit. Then, using a small knife, trim away the beard (the weed caught between the closed shells) and scrape off any barnacles.

2 Place the prepared mussels in a large bowl, cover with *cold* salted water and sprinkle over the oatmeal. Leave in a cool place overnight, then drain and wash well. Check all mussels are still tightly closed.

3 Skin, seed and roughly chop the tomatoes (reserving any juices). Heat the oil in a large saucepan and add the onion, garlic and thyme. Cook, stirring, for 1–2 minutes, then stir in the tomatoes and any juices, the tomato purée, vinegar, cider and salt and pepper to taste. Add the mussels, bring to the boil, cover tightly and cook over a moderate heat for 5–7 minutes, shaking the pan occasionally, until all the mussels have opened.

4 Using a slotted spoon, transfer the mussels to a warmed serving dish, discarding any with unopened shells. Bring the cooking liquor to the boil and boil rapidly for 1–2 minutes or until slightly reduced. Season to taste with salt and pepper. Serve garnished with parsley.

Nutritional analysis	
370 kcals/1545 kJ	14 mg Iron ★ ★ ★ ★
27 g Protein	249 mg Calcium ★ ★ ★
13 g Fat	68 mg Vitamin C ★ ★ ★ ★ ★
29 g Carbohydrate	8.8 mcg Vitamin E ★ ★ ★ ★ ★
6 g Fibre ★	

Stir-Fried Kippers and Cucumber

The mild flavour of the cucumber has a calming effect on the strength of the kippers. Serve with warm wholemeal pitta bread. Kippers contain large amounts of vitamin D and vitamin B_{12}. Food sources of vitamin D are particularly valuable during the winter months when the skin is not exposed to much sunlight. Good body levels of vitamin D are necessary for the absorption of calcium from food.

SERVES 4
450 g (1 lb) naturally smoked kipper fillets
½ cucumber
1 bunch of spring onions, trimmed
15 ml (1 tbsp) polyunsaturated oil
15 ml (1 tbsp) reduced-sodium soya sauce, preferably naturally fermented shoyu
10 ml (2 tsp) lemon juice
10 ml (2 tsp) poppy seeds
pepper

1 Skin the kippers, then cut each fillet diagonally into 2 cm (¾ inch) slices. Cut the cucumber into 4 cm (1½ inch) long thin strips. Cut the spring onions into similar-sized lengths.
2 Heat the oil in a wok or large frying pan, add the onion and cook, stirring, for 2–3 minutes.
3 Add the kipper and cucumber strips and cook for a further minute. Mix in the soy sauce, lemon juice, poppy seeds and pepper to taste. Stir-fry for a further 2–3 minutes or until heated through. Serve immediately.

Nutritional analysis	
190 kcals/785 kJ	6.8 mg Vitamin B$_{12}$ ★ ★ ★ ★ ★
17 g Protein	11 mg Vitamin C ★ ★
12 g Fat	15 mcg Vitamin D ★ ★ ★ ★ ★
3.8 g Carbohydrate	122 mg Calcium ★ ★
1.1 g Fibre	

Omelette Fines Herbes

Only use fresh herbs when making this favourite French dish. Serve with a salad of mixed lettuce dressed with a little nut oil and accompanied by warm French bread. As well as being an excellent source of protein, eggs provide a range of minerals and vitamins.

SERVES 2
4 eggs
15 ml (1 tbsp) chopped fresh chervil
15 ml (1 tbsp) chopped fresh parsley
10 ml (2 tsp) snipped fresh chives
10 ml (2 tsp) chopped fresh thyme
salt and pepper
15 g (½ oz) polyunsaturated margarine

1 In a bowl, whisk together the eggs, herbs, 30 ml (2 tbsp) water and salt and pepper to taste.
2 Heat the margarine in a non-stick frying pan until it just begins to foam. Pour in the egg mixture and stir lightly with a wooden spatula, at the same time gently tilting the pan from side to side to allow the uncooked egg mixture to flow underneath the cooked mixture and set.
3 When the omelette is lightly set, fold it in half, cook for 1 minute, then turn out on to a warmed serving plate. Divide into two portions and serve immediately.

Nutritional analysis	
220 kcals/925 kJ	310 mcg Vitamin A ★ ★
14 g Protein	13 mg Vitamin C ★ ★ ★
18 g Fat	3.8 mcg Vitamin E ★ ★
0.8 g Carbohydrate	2.9 mg Iron ★ ★
0.8 g Fibre	

Mushroom Soufflé

Vitamin B₂ (riboflavin) is found particularly in milk and milk products. Easily destroyed by exposure to ultra-violet light, this vitamin is essential for energy production and oxygen transport. Deficiency results in severe dryness, burning and cracks in the skin.

SERVES 4
200 ml (7 fl oz) semi-skimmed
milk
slices of onion and carrot, 1 bay
leaf and 6 black peppercorns,
for flavouring
40 g (1½ oz) polyunsaturated
margarine

100 g (4 oz) mushrooms, sliced
30 ml (2 tbsp) plain flour
10 ml (2 tsp) Dijon mustard
salt and pepper
cayenne
4 whole eggs, separated
1 extra egg white

1 Grease a 1.3 litre (2¼ pint) soufflé dish.
2 Place the milk in a medium saucepan with the flavouring ingredients. Bring to the boil, remove from the heat, cover, and leave to infuse for 30 minutes. Strain and reserve the milk.
3 Melt the margarine in a medium non-stick saucepan, add the mushrooms, cover and cook for 2–3 minutes or until softened. Stir in the flour, mustard and salt, pepper and cayenne to taste. Cook gently for 1 minute, stirring, then remove from the heat and gradually stir in the milk. Bring to the boil slowly and continue to cook, stirring, until the sauce thickens. Cool a little.
4 Beat the egg yolks into the cooled sauce one at a time. Using a hand or electric mixer, whisk the egg whites until they stand in stiff peaks.
5 Mix one large spoonful of egg white into the sauce to lighten its texture. Gently pour the sauce over the remaining egg whites and fold the ingredients lightly together until the egg whites are just incorporated.
6 Pour the soufflé mixture carefully into the prepared dish and smooth the surface with a palette knife. Place on a baking sheet and cook in the oven at 180°C (350°F) mark 4 for about 30 minutes or until golden brown on the top, well risen and just firm to the touch with a hint of softness in the centre.

Nutritional Analysis	
220 kcals/920 kJ	0.46 mg Vitamin B₂ ★ ★
10 g Protein	3.4 mcg Vitamin E ★ ★
16 g Fat	114 mg Calcium ★ ★
9.1 g Carbohydrate	1.9 mg Iron ★
0.9 g Fibre	

Spinach and Cheese Quiche with Crisp Potato Crust

The large amount of vitamin A in this dish comes from various sources, such as the spinach leaves and milk products. It is essential for maintaining and protecting healthy skin.

SERVES 6

100 g (4 oz) plain wholemeal flour
50 g (2 oz) polyunsaturated margarine
100 g (4 oz) potatoes, scrubbed and finely grated
1 small onion, skinned and grated
salt and pepper
5 ml (1 tsp) polyunsaturated oil
275 g (10 oz) trimmed spinach leaves, finely shredded

3 eggs
225 g (8 oz) ricotta cheese
100 g (4 oz) low-fat soft cheese
30 ml (2 tbsp) freshly grated Parmesan cheese
finely grated rind of 1 lemon
juice of ½ lemon
50 ml (2 fl oz) semi-skimmed milk
freshly grated nutmeg
paprika

1 To make the crust, put the flour in a bowl and rub in the margarine until the mixture resembles fine breadcrumbs. Squeeze the grated potatoes in a cloth to remove as much excess moisture as possible. Add to the flour mixture with the onion and salt and pepper to taste. Mix to a firm dough.

2 With lightly floured fingers, press the dough in a thin even layer over the base and sides of a 20 cm (8 inch) flan tin or dish. Bake at 200°C (400°F) mark 6 for 20 minutes. Brush with the oil and bake for a further 10 minutes or until the crust is cooked through and crisp.

3 Meanwhile, place the spinach in a steamer over boiling water. Cover tightly and steam for 1 minute or until just tender. Set aside.

4 Beat together the eggs, ricotta cheese, low-fat soft cheese, half the Parmesan cheese, the lemon rind and juice and milk until smooth. Add the spinach and mix gently. Season to taste with lots of nutmeg and pepper and a little salt.

5 Reduce the oven to 180°C (350°F) mark 4. Spoon the spinach and cheese mixture into the cooked crust and level the surface. Sprinkle with the remaining Parmesan cheese and a little nutmeg and paprika. Bake for 30–35 minutes or until lightly coloured and set. Serve warm or cold.

Nutritional Analysis	
285 kcals/1190 kJ	608 mcg Vitamin A ★ ★ ★ ★ ★
16 g Protein	17 mg Vitamin C ★ ★ ★
17 g Fat	4.1 mcg Vitamin E ★ ★ ★
19 g Carbohydrate	243 mg Calcium ★ ★ ★
2.4 g Fibre	6.6 mg Iron ★ ★ ★

Aubergine and Bean Gratin

Pulses, such as cannellini beans, are the richest source of vegetable protein and, for this reason, are very valuable in a vegetarian diet. This dish also contains the minerals potassium and calcium, both of which are involved in nerve control.

SERVES 4
2 medium aubergines
15 g (½ oz) polyunsaturated
margarine
1 onion, skinned and chopped
1 garlic clove, skinned and
crushed
100 g (4 oz) button mushrooms

225 g (8 oz) can cannellini
beans, drained and rinsed
2 tomatoes, chopped
pepper
30 ml (2 tbsp) freshly grated
Parmesan cheese
parsley sprigs, to garnish

1 Cut the ends off the aubergines and cook the aubergines in boiling water for about 10 minutes or until tender.
2 Cut the aubergines in half lengthways and scoop out the flesh, leaving 0.5 cm (¼ inch) shells. Finely chop the flesh and reserve the shells.
3 Melt the margarine in a saucepan and add the onion, garlic and chopped aubergine flesh. Cook gently for 5 minutes. Add the mushrooms, beans, tomatoes and pepper to taste.
4 Stuff the aubergine shells with the bean mixture and sprinkle with Parmesan cheese. Place under a hot grill for 4–5 minutes or until heated through. Serve hot, garnished with parsley.

Nutritional Analysis	
145 kcals/600 kJ	24 mg Vitamin C ★
7.4 g Protein	950 mg Potassium ★ ★
5.6 g Fat	136 mg Calcium ★ ★
16 g Carbohydrate	2.2 mg Iron ★
7.2 g Fibre ★ ★	

Goat's Cheese Tarts

These flavoursome savoury tarts contain iron, calcium and vitamin E. Iron is important for the production of red blood cells which supply oxygen to all body cells, including those of the skin.

MAKES 4
50 g (2 oz) plain wholemeal flour
50 g (2 oz) plain flour
salt and pepper
50 g (2 oz) polyunsaturated margarine
1 egg, separated

50 g (2 oz) soft goat's cheese, any coarse rind removed
100 ml (4 fl oz) semi-skimmed milk
8 green and 8 black olives, stoned and chopped
15 ml (1 tbsp) capers, drained

1 Put the flours and a little salt in a bowl and rub in the margarine until the mixture resembles fine breadcrumbs. Add enough water to form a dough. Chill for 30 minutes.
2 Divide the dough into four. Roll out each piece to a round and use to line four 10 cm (4 inch) flan tins or dishes. Prick with a fork and bake blind at 200°C (400°F) mark 6 for 5 minutes. Remove from the oven and lower the oven temperature to 190°C (375°F) mark 5.
3 Meanwhile, beat together the cheese, egg yolk, milk, olives, capers and salt and pepper to taste. Whisk the egg white until stiff and fold into the mixture.
4 Divide the filling between the pastry cases and bake for a further 25 minutes. Serve the tarts warm.

Nutritional Analysis Per Tart	
285 kcals/1200 kJ	186 mcg Vitamin A ★ ★
9.3 g Protein	3.6 mcg Vitamin E ★ ★
19 g Fat	167 mg Calcium ★ ★
21 g Carbohydrate	1.6 mg Iron ★
2.9 g Fibre	

Baked Jacket Potatoes with Hummus

Here is a healthy hummus recipe. You will only need to use half of this quantity to fill the potatoes. Store the remainder in the refrigerator and use as a dip or spread. The skins of potatoes provide a valuable source of insoluble dietary fibre which speeds up the transit of waste material through the digestive system. A disturbed digestive system is reflected in one's skin and eyes.

SERVES 4

425 g (15 oz) can chick-peas, drained and rinsed
30 ml (2 tbsp) olive oil
2 garlic cloves, skinned
grated rind and juice of 1 lemon
30 ml (2 tbsp) tahini
4 potatoes, each weighing about 225 g (8 oz), scrubbed
75 g (3 oz) low-fat soft cheese

1 To make the hummus, place the chick-peas in a blender or food processor with the olive oil, garlic, lemon rind and juice and tahini. Blend until very smooth.
2 Put into a bowl, cover and chill for 2–3 hours to let the flavours develop.
3 Insert a metal skewer into each potato. Place on a baking sheet and cook at 220°C (425°F) mark 7 for 45–50 minutes or until soft and cooked through. Remove the skewers.
4 Stir the cheese into half of the hummus and check the seasoning. Cut a cross in the top of each potato and spoon in the hummus mixture. Serve at once.

Nutritional Analysis	
300 kcals/1250 kJ	33 mg Vitamin C ★ ★ ★ ★ ★
9.5 g Protein	0.57 mg Vitamin B$_6$ ★ ★
8 g Fat	1395 mg Potassium ★ ★ ★
51 g Carbohydrate	2.4 mg Iron ★ ★
6.4 g Fibre ★ ★	

Avocado and Chick-Pea Salad

The combination of Quark and semi-skimmed milk makes a healthy low-fat dressing for this unusual salad. There are large amounts of iron and folic acid in this dish, both of which are required for red blood cell production. The skin relies on healthy blood circulation to provide oxygen and other nutrients.

SERVES 4
45 ml (3 tbsp) lemon juice
50 g (2 oz) natural Quark
100 ml (4 fl oz) semi-skimmed milk
30 ml (2 tbsp) snipped fresh chives or parsley
salt and pepper
1 avocado
450 g (1 lb) fresh young spinach, with stalks removed, finely shredded
100 g (4 oz) radicchio, finely shredded
400 g (14 oz) can chick-peas, drained and rinsed
1 slice of wholemeal bread, toasted and cubed
2 eggs, hard boiled and chopped
paprika

1 To make the dressing, place 30 ml (2 tbsp) lemon juice, the Quark and milk in a bowl and whisk until smooth. Add the herbs, reserving some for garnish, and salt and pepper to taste. Set aside.
2 Peel the avocado, discard the stone and dice. Coat with the remaining lemon juice to prevent discoloration.
3 Mix together the spinach, radicchio, avocado and chick-peas and arrange on a large serving platter.
4 Scatter the toast cubes and egg on top and sprinkle over a little paprika.
5 To serve, spoon a little of the dressing over the salad and garnish with the reserved snipped chives or parsley. Serve the remaining dressing separately.

Nutritional Analysis	
310 kcals/1290 kJ	16 mg Iron ★ ★ ★ ★
15 g Protein	1232 mcg Vitamin A ★ ★ ★ ★ ★
21 g Fat	59 mg Vitamin C ★ ★ ★ ★ ★
17 g Carbohydrate	217 mg Folic Acid ★ ★ ★
6.9 g Fibre ★ ★	

Yogurt Dips with Crudités

Serve these dips with a selection of vegetables that give a good contrast of colour, flavour and texture. The dips provide small amounts of nutrients, particularly calcium, which complement the vitamins and minerals present in the vegetables.

SERVES 4
fresh vegetables, cut into bite-sized pieces, and wholemeal pitta bread, to serve
BLUE CHEESE DIP
150 ml (¼ pint) Greek-style natural yogurt
50 g (2 oz) Danish Blue cheese
1 garlic clove, skinned and crushed
THOUSAND ISLAND DIP
150 ml (¼ pint) Greek-style natural yogurt

10 ml (2 tsp) tomato purée
10 ml (2 tsp) creamed horseradish sauce
CONTINENTAL DIP
150 ml (¼ pint) Greek-style natural yogurt
1 pickled gherkin, chopped
30 ml (2 tbsp) chopped fresh parsley
6 stuffed olives, finely chopped

To make the dips, mix together the ingredients for each one in individual bowls. Chill for at least 20 minutes, preferably up to 2 hours. Serve with fresh vegetables and wholemeal pitta bread.

Nutritional analysis Blue Cheese	
95 kcals/395 kJ	1.8 g Carbohydrate
5.2 g Protein	0 g Fibre
7.4 g Fat	118 mg Calcium ★ ★
Thousand Island	
60 kcals/240 kJ	2.2 g Carbohydrate
2.5 g Protein	0 g Fibre
4.4 g Fat	48 mg Calcium
Continental	
60 kcals/240 kJ	1.0 Fibre
2.7 g Protein	12 mg Vitamin C ★ ★
4.6 g Fat	76 mg Calcium ★
1.6 g Carbohydrate	

5

Fish Main Dishes

Fish is one of the most nutritious foods available since it is high in protein, vitamins and minerals and relatively low in calories. Oily fish, in particular, is a rich source of vitamin D and certain 'essential fatty acids' which appear to be of benefit to people suffering from psoriasis. There are recipes here for family meals and for entertaining, all so tempting that you will want to include fish often in your diet. They need only simple accompaniments such as brown rice, a salad, or lightly cooked vegetables.

Mediterranean Fish Stew

Serve with lots of crusty wholemeal bread to soak up the delicious juices. Potassium is required for maintaining normal water balance within body cells. Low intakes result in tissue swelling (oedema).

SERVES 4
12 fresh mussels
30 ml (2 tbsp) olive oil
1 onion, skinned and thinly sliced
1 garlic clove, skinned and crushed
450 g (1 lb) tomatoes, skinned, seeded and chopped
300 ml (½ pint) dry white wine
450 ml (¾ pint) fish stock
15 ml (1 tbsp) chopped fresh dill or 5 ml (1 tsp) dillweed

10 ml (2 tsp) chopped fresh rosemary or 5 ml (1 tsp) dried
15 ml (1 tbsp) tomato purée
salt and pepper
450 g (1 lb) monkfish fillet, skinned and cut into large chunks
4 jumbo prawns, peeled
225 g (8 oz) squid, cleaned and cut into rings
chopped fresh parsley, to garnish

1 To clean the mussels, put them in a large bowl and scrape well under cold running water. Discard any that are open. Rinse until there is no trace of sand in the bowl.
2 Heat the oil in a large saucepan or flameproof casserole and gently cook the onion for 3–4 minutes. Add the garlic and tomatoes and cook for a further 3–4 minutes.
3 Add the white wine, stock, herbs, tomato purée and salt and pepper to taste and bring to the boil. Lower the heat and simmer for a further 5 minutes.
4 Add the monkfish and simmer for 5 minutes. Add the prawns and squid and simmer for a further 5 minutes. Add the prepared mussels, cover the pan and cook for 3–4 minutes or until the shells open. Discard any mussels that do not open. Ladle the stew into individual bowls, sprinkle with parsley and serve.

Nutritional analysis	
320 kcals/1330 kJ	25 mg Vitamin C ★ ★ ★ ★
36 g Protein	852 mg Potassium ★ ★
11 g Fat	4.3 mg Iron ★ ★
5.9 g Carbohydrate	1.7 mg Zinc ★
1.8 g Fibre	

Monkfish in a Rich Tomato Sauce

The firm texture of monkfish is perfect for casseroles as it doesn't disintegrate on cooking. Tomatoes and dark green leafy vegetables and herbs, eg parsley, contribute vitamin A, which helps protect the skin against sunburn. Tomatoes are also valuable for their potassium content.

SERVES 4
900 g (2 lb) monkfish
30 ml (2 tbsp) olive oil
15 ml (1 tbsp) lemon juice
5 ml (1 tsp) dried oregano
450 g (1 lb) ripe tomatoes
1 medium onion, skinned and chopped
1 garlic clove, skinned and crushed

15 ml (1 tbsp) plain flour
15 ml (1 tbsp) tomato purée
12 green olives, halved and stoned
50 ml (2 fl oz) dry vermouth
salt and pepper
30 ml (2 tbsp) chopped fresh parsley

1 Skin the monkfish, then remove the flesh from the bone and cut into 2.5 cm (1 inch) chunks. Place in a bowl with half the oil, the lemon juice and oregano. Stir gently, then cover and leave to marinate for about 2 hours.

2 Meanwhile, skin, seed and roughly chop the tomatoes, reserving any juice.

3 Heat the remaining oil in a large frying pan, add the onion and garlic and cook for 1–2 minutes. Stir in the flour and cook for a further minute.

4 Add the tomatoes (and any juice), the tomato purée, olives, dry vermouth and 50 ml (2 fl oz) water. Bring to the boil, stirring all the time, then boil for 1 minute only.

5 Gently stir in the fish and marinade. Cover and cook over a moderate heat for about 20 minutes or until the fish is just tender. Season to taste with salt and pepper, then stir in the parsley.

Nutritional analysis	
315 kcals/1310 kJ	1069 mg Potassium ★ ★
35 g Protein	2.4 mg Iron ★ ★
13 g Fat	222 mcg Vitamin A ★
9.8 g Carbohydrate	43 mg Vitamin C ★ ★ ★ ★ ★
3.7 g Fibre ★	

Lemon Sole in Lettuce

Niacin is a B vitamin required for energy production from proteins, fats and carbohydrates. It is also essential for maintaining a healthy skin and digestive tract.

SERVES 4
8 large lettuce leaves, thick stalks removed
8 lemon sole fillets, each weighing about 100 g (4 oz), skinned
15 ml (1 tbsp) lemon juice
salt and pepper
100 g (4 oz) cooked peeled prawns
15 ml (1 tbsp) chopped fresh dill
150 ml (¼ pint) fish stock or dry white wine
lemon slices, to garnish

1 Drop the lettuce leaves into a large saucepan of boiling water and simmer for 2 minutes. Drain and quickly cool in cold water. Drain again and dry on absorbent kitchen paper, then spread out on a flat surface.
2 Sprinkle the fillets with a little of the lemon juice and salt and pepper to taste. Arrange a few prawns in the centre of each fillet and sprinkle over half the dill. Fold the fish into thirds to enclose the prawns.
3 Place each folded fillet on a lettuce leaf and roll up again, folding the edges in to form a neat parcel.
4 Place the fish parcels in a non-stick frying pan and sprinkle over the remaining lemon juice, stock or wine and pepper to taste. Cover and cook gently for 15 minutes or until tender.
5 Transfer the fish to a warmed serving dish. Boil the cooking juices until reduced to about 90 ml (6 tbsp). Stir in the remaining dill and pour over the fish. Serve garnished with lemon slices.

Nutritional analysis	
220 kcals/930 kJ	24 mg Vitamin C ★ ★ ★
40 g Protein	107 mg Calcium ★ ★
3.4 g Fat	1.9 mg Iron ★
1.6 g Carbohydrate	7.4 mg Niacin ★ ★ ★
1.6 g Fibre	

Bass Baked in Mint

This is a wonderful dish to make at the height of summer, when you have an abundance of mint in the garden. It contains substantial amounts of vitamin B_{12}, a vitamin that is vital to the production of new blood cells. B_{12} can be stored in the body and, as it is needed only in very small amounts, a deficiency is rare. As the prime sources are meat, fish and dairy products, vegans may risk developing such a deficiency.

SERVES 4
900 g (2 lb) sea bass, scaled and gutted
salt and pepper
polyunsaturated oil
2 handfuls of mint sprigs
150 ml (¼ pint) dry white wine
1 medium onion, skinned and finely chopped
15 ml (1 tbsp) orange juice
60 ml (4 tbsp) whipping cream
mint sprigs and orange slices, to garnish

1 Lightly season the fish inside and out with salt and pepper. Brush a baking dish with a little oil, scatter over half the mint and lay the fish on it. Stuff some more mint inside the fish and scatter the rest over the top.
2 Pour over the dry white wine and sprinkle with the finely chopped onion and the orange juice.
3 Cover with kitchen foil and bake at 180°C (350°F) mark 4 for 30–35 minutes or until the fish is just cooked. Keep warm.
4 Strain the cooking juices into a saucepan and boil rapidly until they are reduced by half. Reduce the heat and stir in the cream. Check the seasoning.
5 Pour the sauce over the fish and garnish with mint and orange.

Nutritional analysis	
260 kcals/1095 kJ	6.3 mg Vitamin B_{12} ★ ★ ★ ★ ★
30 g Protein	13 mg Vitamin C ★ ★ ★
10 g Fat	2.2 mcg Vitamin E ★ ★
4.4 g Carbohydrate	1.8 mg Iron ★
0.8 g Fibre	

Spiced Mackerel

The spices in this dish enhance the flavour of the food so that it is unnecessary to add salt. Although high in fat, mackerel, like other oily fish, contains essential fatty acids, particularly those of the Omega-3 series. These fatty acids, in conjunction with large amounts of vitamin D, have been found to assist in the healing of wounds and burns.

SERVES 4

4 whole fresh mackerel, each weighing 350–450 g (12 oz–1 lb), cleaned
200 ml (7 fl oz) low-fat natural yogurt
finely grated rind and juice of 1 lemon
1–2 garlic cloves, skinned and chopped
a few sprigs of fresh coriander

5 cm (2 inch) piece of fresh root ginger, skinned and crushed, or 5 ml (1 tsp) ground ginger
10 ml (2 tsp) cumin seeds
5 ml (1 tsp) fenugreek seeds
5 ml (1 tsp) ground turmeric
2.5–5 ml (½–1 tsp) chilli powder
lemon wedges and fresh coriander sprigs, to garnish

1 Make deep, diagonal slashes on both sides of each mackerel, then arrange the fish side by side in a dish.

2 Put the yogurt, lemon rind and juice, garlic, coriander, ginger, cumin seeds, fenugreek seeds, turmeric and chilli powder in a blender or food processor and blend to a thin paste. Pour over the mackerel, turning the fish to coat them. Loosely cover and leave to marinate in a cool place for 1–4 hours.

3 Put the fish on a rack in the grill pan and cook under a medium grill for about 15 minutes or until the flesh flakes easily when tested with a fork. Turn the fish over once during cooking and brush with any remaining marinade in the dish. Lift the fish carefully on to a warmed serving platter and garnish with lemon wedges and coriander sprigs. Serve hot.

Nutritional analysis	
645 kcals/2690 kJ	1.9 mg Vitamin B₆ ★ ★ ★ ★ ★
54 g Protein	27 mg Vitamin B₁₂ ★ ★ ★ ★ ★
45 g Fat	47 mcg Vitamin D ★ ★ ★ ★ ★
5.4 g Carbohydrate	6.6 mg Iron ★ ★ ★
0.7 g Fibre	

Mackerel Fillets in Oatmeal and Almonds

Herrings could replace the mackerel in this recipe but keep the weight the same. Serve with a watercress and orange salad. Oily fish like mackerel should figure frequently in the diet. The type of fat in them contains essential fatty acids which benefit not only the skin but the blood circulatory system as well.

SERVES 4
2 whole mackerel, each
weighing about 550 g
(1 ¼ lb) cleaned
30 ml (2 tbsp) seasoned flour

75 g (3 oz) whole almonds
100 g (4 oz) coarse oatmeal
1 egg, beaten
60 ml (4 tbsp) orange juice

1 Cut the heads off the mackerel, then, using a sharp knife, slit the fish open all the way along the underside.

2 Place the fish, flesh-side down, on a board and press firmly all along the backbone to loosen the bone and flatten the fish. Turn the fish flesh-side up and ease out the bones.

3 Cut each fish in half to give two fillets, then, if wished, carefully skin each one. (This may be difficult if the fish is really fresh.) Coat each fillet lightly in the flour.

4 Blanch the almonds in boiling water for about 1 minute. Pop out of the skins and chop finely. Place in a shallow dish with the oatmeal.

5 Dip each mackerel fillet into the beaten egg, then coat in the nuts and oatmeal. Place on a baking sheet.

6 Sprinkle a little orange juice over each fillet, then cook under a hot grill for about 5 minutes on each side. Serve immediately.

Nutritional analysis	
525 kcals/2195 kJ	17 mg Vitamin C ★ ★ ★
30 g Protein	19 mcg Vitamin D ★ ★ ★ ★ ★
32 g Fat	4.3 mcg Vitamin E ★ ★ ★
32 g Carbohydrate	2.4 mg Zinc ★
5.8 g Fibre ★	

Stuffed Sea Trout

This simple stuffed trout is cooked in wine in a parcel of foil so the cooked fish is succulent and tender. It contains a significant amount of iron, helping to avoid anaemia, one of the first signs of which is dull, 'ashy' facial skin.

SERVES 4
25 g (1 oz) polyunsaturated margarine
½ small onion, skinned and finely chopped
1 small fennel bulb, trimmed and finely chopped
1 garlic clove, skinned and crushed
50 g (2 oz) fresh wholemeal breadcrumbs

50 g (2 oz) flaked almonds, toasted and finely chopped
grated rind and juice of ½ lemon
salt and pepper
1.4 kg (3 lb) sea trout, cleaned and boned, with head removed
75 ml (3 fl oz) dry white wine

1 To make the stuffing, melt the margarine in a non-stick frying pan and cook the onion, fennel and garlic for about 5 minutes or until soft. Stir in the breadcrumbs, almonds, lemon rind and juice and season to taste with salt and pepper.
2 Open out the fish and spread the stuffing evenly along one side. Fold over the other half of the fish and put on a lightly greased piece of kitchen foil large enough to enclose the fish. Pour the wine over and seal the foil edges together. Carefully transfer to a roasting tin.
3 Cook at 190°C (375°F) mark 5 for 35–40 minutes or until the fish is cooked through and the flesh flakes easily when tested with a fork. Open out the foil and carefully transfer the fish to a serving dish. Pour over any cooking juices and serve.

Nutritional analysis	
415 kcals/1745 kJ	4.1 mcg Vitamin E ★ ★ ★
48 g Protein	909 mg Potassium ★ ★
21 g Fat	115 mg Calcium ★ ★
7.1 g Carbohydrate	3 mg Iron ★ ★
3.2 g Fibre ★	

Sardines with Lime and Herbs

This easy-to-prepare sardine dish is high in vitamin D and also provides calcium. Calcium is dependent on a good body status of vitamin D for its absorption and metabolism.

SERVES 4
900 g (2 lb) fresh sardines (at least 12), cleaned if wished
60 ml (4 tbsp) chopped mixed fresh herbs, such as mint, parsley, sage

finely grated rind and juice of 2 limes
30 ml (2 tbsp) olive oil
salt and pepper
fresh herbs and lemon wedges, to garnish

1 Wash the sardines well. Mix together the herbs, lime rind and juice, oil, and salt and pepper to taste.
2 Grill the sardines for 5–7 minutes each side, basting with the herb dressing. Serve immediately or leave in the dressing to cool completely.
3 Garnish with herbs and lemon wedges before serving.

Nutritional analysis	
235 kcals/985 kJ	28 mg Vitamin C ★ ★ ★ ★ ★
27 g Protein	1.3 mg Vitamin B_6 ★ ★ ★
14 g Fat	10 mcg Vitamin D ★ ★ ★ ★ ★
0.2 g Carbohydrate	5.1 mg Iron ★ ★ ★
1.4 g Fibre	4.1 mg Zinc ★ ★

Curried Fish with Coconut

Coley can sometimes look rather grey but the colour is cleverly disguised in this mildly spiced sauce. More than half the recommended daily amount of vitamin E is present in each portion. Vitamin E has a number of protective roles and also acts as a diuretic, preventing excess fluid retention and puffy skin.

SERVES 4
900 g (2 lb) coley fillet
20 ml (4 tsp) seasoned flour
75 g (3 oz) creamed coconut
450 g (1 lb) ripe tomatoes
30 ml (2 tbsp) polyunsaturated oil
1 medium onion, skinned and chopped

1 garlic clove, skinned and crushed
2.5 ml (½ tsp) each ground coriander, cumin and turmeric
30 ml (2 tbsp) chopped fresh coriander
salt and pepper
lime wedges and fresh coriander, to garnish

1 Rinse the fish, pat dry on absorbent kitchen paper, then carefully skin each fillet. Cut into large pieces and coat lightly in seasoned flour.

2 Break up the creamed coconut and dissolve in 150 ml (¼ pint) boiling water, stirring well.

3 Skin, halve and seed the tomatoes, then chop the flesh into large pieces. Push the juices through a nylon sieve and reserve.

4 Heat the oil in a large frying pan, add the onion, garlic, spices and fresh coriander and cook, stirring, for 2–3 minutes. Stir in the tomato flesh and juices, the coconut solution and salt and pepper to taste and cook for a further minute.

5 Remove from the heat and gently stir in the fish, taking care not to break up the flesh. Return the pan to a gentle heat and cook, covered, for about 12 minutes or until the fish is just cooked and beginning to flake. Check the seasoning. Garnish with lime wedges and fresh coriander leaves.

Nutritional analysis	
490 kcals/2040 kJ	54 mg Vitamin C ★ ★ ★ ★ ★
42 g Protein	6 mcg Vitamin E ★ ★ ★
31 g Fat	1263 mg Potassium ★ ★ ★
12 g Carbohydrate	5 mg Iron ★ ★ ★
4.3 g Fibre ★	

Haddock and Prawn Stir-Fry

Stir-frying is fast and healthy. It uses little oil and fewer vitamins are lost during cooking. This stir-fried dish therefore retains more nutrients than if it were cooked by a slower method.

SERVES 4
225 g (8 oz) can pineapple slices in natural juice, drained, with juice reserved
15 ml (1 tbsp) reduced-sodium soy sauce, preferably naturally fermented shoyu
60 ml (4 tbsp) malt vinegar
30 ml (2 tbsp) light muscovado sugar
15 ml (1 tbsp) tomato purée
30 ml (2 tbsp) dry sherry
30 ml (2 tbsp) cornflour
45 ml (3 tbsp) polyunsaturated oil
450 g (1 lb) haddock fillet, skinned and cut into bite-sized pieces
1 small onion, skinned and sliced
1 red pepper, cored, seeded and thinly sliced

2 carrots, scrubbed and sliced
2.5 cm (1 inch) piece of fresh
root ginger, peeled and chopped
225 g (8 oz) can water
chestnuts, drained and sliced

100 g (4 oz) button mushrooms,
sliced
225 g (8 oz) fresh bean sprouts
175 g (6 oz) cooked peeled
prawns, thawed if frozen

1 Cut each pineapple slice into chunks. Make up the reserved juice
to 300 ml (½ pint) with water. Add the soy sauce, vinegar, sugar,
tomato purée, sherry and cornflour. Mix until smooth.
2 Heat 15 ml (1 tbsp) oil in a large non-stick frying pan or wok. Add
the haddock and stir-fry for about 5 minutes or until just cooked.
Transfer to a plate and keep hot.
3 Add the remaining oil to the pan and cook the onion, pepper,
carrots and ginger over a high heat for 3 minutes, stirring constantly. Add the pineapple, water chestnuts and mushrooms and
stir-fry for a further 2 minutes. Stir the pineapple juice mixture
and add to the pan. Bring to the boil, stirring. Add the bean sprouts,
prawns and haddock and heat through. Serve at once.

Nutritional analysis	
395 kcals/1645 kJ	736 mcg Vitamin A ★ ★ ★ ★ ★
33 g Protein	66 mg Vitamin C ★ ★ ★ ★ ★
13 g Fat	6.4 mcg Vitamin E ★ ★ ★ ★
36 g Carbohydrate	3.6 mg Iron ★ ★
3.3 g Fibre ★	

Fish in Filo Pastry

*Filo pastry is time-consuming and fairly difficult to make. Ready-
made filo pastry is available from good delicatessens and large
supermarkets. Filo pastry dishes are usually very high in fat. The
fat content of this one, however, makes up only 13 per cent of the
total kcal/kJ (energy) content.*

SERVES 4
8 white fish fillets, such as sole
or plaice, each weighing about
75 g (3 oz), skinned and cut into
thin strips
30 ml (2 tbsp) lemon or lime
juice

3 courgettes, trimmed and
grated
2 shallots, skinned and chopped
salt and pepper
8 sheets of filo pastry

1 Lightly grease a baking sheet. In a bowl, combine the fish, juice, courgettes and shallots. Add salt and pepper to taste, mix well, then divide into eight equal portions.

2 Work with one sheet of filo pastry at a time, keeping the remainder covered with a damp cloth. Fold the filo in half lengthways. Place one-eighth of the fish mixture in one corner and pat out lightly. Fold the filo over the filling at right angles to make a triangle. Continue folding the filo strip over to form a neat triangular-shaped parcel. Repeat with the remaining filo and fish mixture.

3 Arrange the eight parcels on the baking sheet. Cook at 190°C (375°F) mark 5 for 25 minutes or until golden and cooked through. If necessary, cover the pointed ends of the parcels with kitchen foil during cooking to prevent over-browning. Serve hot.

Nutritional analysis	
270 kcals/1130 kJ	8.8 mg Vitamin C ★ ★
30 g Protein	536 mg Potassium ★
3.8 g Fat	1.9 mg Iron ★
31 g Carbohydrate	1.4 mg Zinc ★
1.5 g Fibre	

Salade Niçoise

Olive oil is a mono-unsaturated oil, once thought to play no role in heart disease but now recognised as playing a positive part in its prevention.

SERVES 4
198 g (7 oz) can tuna fish, drained
225 g (8 oz) tomatoes, quartered
50 g (2 oz) black olives, stoned
½ small cucumber, thinly sliced
225 g (8 oz) cooked French beans
2 eggs, hard-boiled, shelled and quartered
15 ml (1 tbsp) chopped fresh parsley
15 ml (1 tbsp) chopped fresh basil
45 ml (3 tbsp) olive oil
30 ml (2 tbsp) lemon juice
1 garlic clove, skinned and crushed
salt and pepper
8 anchovy fillets, halved and drained

1 Flake the tuna into fairly large chunks and mix in a salad bowl with the tomatoes, olives, cucumber slices, beans and eggs.
2 Whisk together the herbs, oil, lemon juice, garlic and salt and pepper to taste, then pour over the salad.
3 Arrange the anchovy fillets in a lattice pattern over the salad and leave to stand for 30 minutes before serving.

Nutritional analysis	
235 kcals/985 kJ	183 mcg Vitamin A ★ ★
18 g Protein	26 mg Vitamin C ★ ★ ★ ★ ★
17 g Fat	4.6 mcg Vitamin E ★ ★ ★
3.2 g Carbohydrate	2.3 mg Iron ★
3.7 g Fibre	

Mixed Seafood Salad

Shellfish is an excellent source of minerals, including zinc. Zinc deficiency becomes apparent with the development of stretch marks on the skin and white spots on fingernails.

SERVES 4
75 g (3 oz) fresh cockles, or 150 g (5 oz) bottled cockles, drained
75 g (3 oz) scallops, halved or quartered
15 ml (1 tbsp) lemon juice
45 ml (3 tbsp) mayonnaise
30 ml (2 tbsp) low-fat natural yogurt
5 ml (1 tsp) grated fresh or bottled horseradish
pepper
75 g (3 oz) cooked peeled prawns
100 g (4 oz) cooked fresh white crab meat, flaked, or 175 g (6 oz) canned crab meat, drained and flaked
100 g (4 oz) black grapes, seeded
1 tomato, finely chopped
a few mixed lettuce leaves

1 If using fresh cockles, rinse them well under cold water, then soak for 2–3 hours. Gently heat them in a saucepan with just a little water, shaking the pan, for about 5 minutes or until the shells open. Remove the cockles from their shells and cook for a further 4 minutes. Drain and set aside to cool.
2 Meanwhile, in another small saucepan, cook the scallops in the lemon juice for 4–5 minutes or until tender. Drain and cool.

3 Mix together the mayonnaise, yogurt, horseradish and pepper to taste. Stir in the scallops, cockles, prawns, crab meat and grapes. Mix lightly together, then fold in the tomato.
4 Place the lettuce on a serving dish and pile the seafood salad on top. Serve at once.

Nutritional analysis	
180 kcals/750 kJ	7 mg Iron ★ ★ ★
18 g Protein	141 mg Calcium ★ ★
9.9 g Fat	2.6 mg Zinc ★ ★
4.5 g Carbohydrate	7.9 mg Vitamin C ★ ★
0.5 g Fibre	

Smoked Mackerel and New Potato Salad

Oily fish contain valuable 'essential fatty acids', particularly those of the Omega-3 series which appear to be of benefit to psoriasis sufferers.

SERVES 4
450 g (1 lb) small new potatoes
60 ml (4 tbsp) apple juice
30 ml (2 tbsp) white wine vinegar
30 ml (2 tbsp) creamed horseradish
salt and pepper

½ cucumber
450 g (1 lb) naturally smoked mackerel fillets
1 red-skinned eating apple
60 ml (4 tbsp) low-fat natural yogurt
shredded lettuce, to serve (optional)

1 Cook the potatoes in boiling salted water for 15–20 minutes or until tender. Meanwhile, whisk together the apple juice, vinegar, horseradish and salt and pepper to taste. Drain the potatoes, halve if necessary, then while still warm stir into the dressing. Leave to cool, stirring occasionally.
2 Meanwhile, cut the cucumber into small chunks. Place in a colander, sprinkle with salt and leave to stand for about 20 minutes. Rinse the cucumber, drain and pat dry with absorbent kitchen paper.
3 Divide the mackerel into coarse flakes, discarding the skin. Core and roughly chop the apple.
4 Gently mix all the ingredients together, including the yogurt,

taking care not to break up the fish. Serve alone or on a bed of shredded lettuce.

Nutritional Analysis	
425 kcals/1785 kJ	26 mg Vitamin C ★ ★ ★ ★ ★
25 g Protein	0.27 mg Vitamin B₁ ★ ★
24 g Fat	1.1 mg Vitamin B₆ ★ ★ ★
29 g Carbohydrate	952 mg Potassium ★ ★
3.1 g Fibre ★	

6

Meat and Poultry Main Dishes

When cooking meat, it is important to remove as much visible fat as possible. Poultry is relatively low in fat, especially if the skin has been removed. Home-made meat and poultry stocks should also be skimmed to remove fat before adding to a recipe. As well as meat and poultry dishes for entertaining, you will find several family-meal ideas in this chapter, including iron-rich liver and kidney recipes which should be incorporated weekly into family meals.

Rack of Lamb in a Herb Overcoat

This crunchy herb crust also works well on a leg or shoulder of lamb, but you need to make double the quantity. Serve it with creamy Potato and Garlic Purée (page 177) and a leafy green vegetable. Red meat, such as lamb, contributes valuable amounts of iron and zinc. Amongst other things, zinc helps the healing of wounds. It is often incorporated in skin salves.

SERVES 4

700 g (1½ lb) best end neck of lamb, chined and trimmed of excess fat
10 ml (2 tsp) whole grain mustard
10 ml (2 tsp) polyunsaturated oil
10 ml (2 tsp) chopped fresh rosemary
10 ml (2 tsp) chopped fresh thyme
30 ml (2 tbsp) chopped fresh parsley
60 ml (4 tbsp) fresh wholemeal breadcrumbs
salt and pepper
200 ml (7 fl oz) red wine

1 Wipe the lamb and place in a roasting tin. Mix together the mustard, oil, herbs, breadcrumbs and salt and pepper to taste. Carefully press this mixture over the fat of the lamb to cover.
2 Place a sheet of kitchen foil loosely over the meat. Roast at 190°C (375°F) mark 5 for about 45 minutes, removing the foil for the last 15 minutes.
3 Transfer the meat to a warm serving plate and keep warm. Drain off any excess fat from the tin, then add the red wine, scraping down the sediment and stirring well. Bring to the boil and simmer for about 5 minutes or until the liquid is reduced by about one-third. Add salt and pepper to taste.
4 To serve, cut the lamb down into chops and pour a little sauce over each.

Nutritional analysis	
230 kcals/965 kJ	11 mg Vitamin C ★ ★
19 g Protein	422 mg Potassium ★
11 g Fat	2.9 mg Iron ★ ★
7.1 g Carbohydrate	2.9 mg Zinc ★ ★
2 g Fibre	

Lamb Tagine

A tagine is a stew of Moroccan origin. There are various types of tagine, many of which contain fruit and aromatic spices. Lamb is naturally high in fat and cholesterol, a potentially harmful constituent of all saturated fats. Chronically elevated blood cholesterol levels can lead to heart disease. However, the fibre present in dried fruit, for example, helps prevent an excessive rise in blood cholesterol levels.

SERVES 6
900 g (2 lb) boned lean lamb, trimmed of fat and cut into large cubes
1.25 ml (¼ tsp) salt
1 onion, skinned and sliced
10 ml (2 tsp) ground coriander
2.5 ml (½ tsp) saffron threads
1 cinnamon stick
5 ml (1 tsp) ground ginger

2.5 ml (½ tsp) ground cumin
juice of 1 lemon
450 g (1 lb) mixed dried fruit, such as prunes, apples, pears and apricots, rinsed, soaked overnight and drained
45 ml (3 tbsp) clear honey
25 g (1 oz) toasted sesame seeds

1 Put the lamb, salt, onion, coriander, saffron, cinnamon stick, ginger, cumin and lemon juice in a heavy-based saucepan. Pour over about 450 ml (¾ pint) water, or just enough to cover the lamb. Cover tightly with a well-fitting lid and simmer over a very low heat for 2 hours.
2 Add the fruit and honey and continue to cook, uncovered, for 20 minutes. Remove the lamb and fruit with a slotted spoon. Skim off any fat, then boil the liquid until reduced to about 150 ml (¼ pint). Discard the cinnamon stick.
3 Return the lamb and fruit to the pan and heat through. Serve hot, sprinkled with the sesame seeds.

Nutritional analysis	
435 kcals/1815 kJ	268 mcg Vitamin A ★ ★ ★
35 g Protein	1551 mg Potassium ★ ★ ★
16 g Fat	7.8 mg Iron ★ ★ ★ ★
41 g Carbohydrate	6.5 mg Zinc ★ ★ ★
14 g Fibre ★ ★ ★	

Beef Burgundy

This rich flavoursome beef casserole needs only plain vegetables or rice to accompany it. Removing all visible traces of fat from the meat and strictly measuring the oil used produces a dramatic reduction in the overall fat content. Present-day dietary recommendations for optimum health suggest that we should eat less fatty foods while the main source of energy should be starchy carbohydrates.

SERVES 4

10 ml (2 tsp) olive oil
550 g (1¼ lb) beef topside, trimmed of all fat and cubed
15 g (½ oz) plain wholemeal flour
30 ml (2 tbsp) brandy
1 onion, skinned and coarsely chopped
2 carrots, scrubbed and sliced
1 garlic clove, skinned and crushed
pepper
1 bouquet garni
150 ml (¼ pint) red Burgundy
150 ml (¼ pint) beef stock (optional)
225 g (8 oz) baby onions, skinned
225 g (8 oz) button mushrooms
lemon juice

1 Brush a heavy-based frying pan with 5 ml (1 tsp) of the oil and heat. Toss the beef in the flour, add to the pan and cook over a medium heat for about 1 minute to seal.

2 Remove the pan from the heat, pour the brandy over and, holding the pan at a safe distance, ignite the brandy. When the flame dies down, add the chopped onion, carrots, garlic, pepper to taste and the bouquet garni. Stir for 1 minute, add the wine and heat gradually. When the mixture begins to bubble, pour into an ovenproof casserole with a tight-fitting lid. The contents should be covered by liquid, so add the stock if necessary.

3 Cover and cook at 150°C (300°F) mark 2 for 1½ hours.

4 Brush the frying pan with the remaining oil, add the baby onions and cook until browned. Add to the casserole and cook for a further 30 minutes. Add the mushrooms and cook for a further 15 minutes. Add lemon juice to taste, remove the bouquet garni and serve.

Nutritional analysis	
290 kcals/1210 kJ	700 mcg Vitamin A ★ ★ ★ ★ ★
31 g Protein	15 mg Vitamin C ★ ★ ★
9.4 g Fat	4.5 mg Iron ★ ★
10 g Carbohydrate	6.2 mg Zinc ★ ★ ★
3.8 g Fibre ★	

Beef Braised in Beer

One portion of this beef braise, which is a meal in itself, contains more than half the recommended daily amount of iron and zinc.

SERVES 6
30 ml (2 tbsp) plain wholemeal flour
2.5 ml (½ tsp) dried mixed herbs
salt and pepper
1.1–1.4 kg (2½–3 lb) lean topside of beef, well trimmed
15 ml (1 tbsp) polyunsaturated oil
2 onions, skinned and quartered
3 potatoes, scrubbed and quartered
2 carrots, scrubbed and cut into large pieces
2 celery sticks, trimmed and cut into large pieces
1 turnip, peeled and cut into bite-sized pieces
1.25 ml (¼ tsp) freshly grated nutmeg
1 bay leaf
150 ml (¼ pint) pale ale

1 Mix together the flour, herbs and salt and pepper to taste. Use to coat the beef. Heat the oil in a flameproof casserole and cook the beef over a fairly high heat for about 5 minutes or until browned all over. Remove from the casserole and set aside.

2 Add the vegetables to the casserole and cook for 3–4 minutes, stirring frequently. Stir any remaining seasoned flour into the casserole, then place the beef on top of the vegetables. Add the nutmeg, bay leaf and pale ale. Cover tightly and cook at 180°C (350°F) mark 4, allowing 45 minutes per 450 g (1 lb) of meat.

3 To serve, lift the meat and vegetables on to a warmed serving dish. Discard the bay leaf and skim the fat from the cooking liquid. Pour a little of the liquid over the meat and vegetables, and serve the remainder separately.

Nutritional analysis	
335 kcals/1405 kJ	467 mcg Vitamin A ★ ★ ★ ★
40 g Protein	17 mg Vitamin C ★ ★ ★
11 g Fat	4.7 mg Iron ★ ★
19 g Carbohydrate	8.3 mg Zinc ★ ★ ★ ★
3.2 g Fibre ★	

Cold Spiced Pork with Nectarine

This would make an attractive buffet party dish to serve with a variety of salads. It contains vitamins B_1 (thiamin), B_3 (niacin) and B_{12}, all of which have their part to play in the building and maintenance of healthy skin.

SERVES 4
30 ml (2 tbsp) clear honey
45 ml (3 tbsp) reduced-sodium
soy sauce, preferably naturally
fermented shoyu
pinch of Chinese five-spice
powder (optional)

450 g (1 lb) pork fillet, trimmed
of excess fat
1 ripe nectarine
watercress, to garnish

1 For the marinade, mix together the honey, soy sauce and five-spice powder, if using. Place the pork in a dish, pour over the marinade and rub it well into the meat. Leave to marinate for 1 hour, turning occasionally.

2 Place the pork on a wire rack over a roasting tin half filled with hot water. Roast at 180°C (350°F) mark 4 for 20 minutes. Turn the meat over, brush with more marinade, then return to the oven for 20 minutes or until the meat is tender. Set the meat aside to cool.

3 Thinly slice the pork. Halve, stone and thinly slice the nectarine. Arrange the pork and nectarine slices alternately, radiating from the centre of a serving dish. Garnish with watercress.

Nutritional analysis	
210 kcals/885 kJ	1 mg Vitamin B_1 ★ ★ ★ ★ ★
24 g Protein	7.4 mg Niacin ★ ★
8.1 g Fat	0.51 mg Vitamin B_6 ★ ★
11 g Carbohydrate	3.4 mg Vitamin B_{12} ★ ★ ★ ★ ★
0.9 g Fibre	2.8 mg Zinc ★ ★

Apricot and Redcurrant Stuffed Pork

Pork is a very good source of vitamin B_1 (thiamin), required for energy production from carbohydrates. Thiamin deficiency can lead to various ailments, such as fatigue, loss of appetite and digestive upsets.

SERVES 4
25 g (1 oz) brown rice
100 g (4 oz) no-soak dried apricots, rinsed and chopped
550–700 g (1¼–1½ lb) pork fillet
½ small onion, skinned and chopped
50 g (2 oz) redcurrants, strung

100 g (4 oz) cooking apple, peeled, cored and chopped
finely grated rind and juice of 1 small orange
30 ml (2 tbsp) chopped fresh parsley
salt and pepper

1 Put the rice and apricots in 150 ml (¼ pint) boiling water. Reduce the heat, cover and simmer for 30 minutes or until just tender and the liquid has been absorbed.
2 Meanwhile, split open the pork fillet lengthways, without cutting it in half. Spread the meat out flat, cut side down, cover with greaseproof paper and pound with a flat mallet to form a 30 × 20 cm (12 × 8 inch) rectangle.
3 Put the onion in a bowl with the redcurrants, apple, orange rind, 15 ml (1 tbsp) chopped parsley, apricots and rice. Add salt and pepper to taste and mix well.
4 Spoon the stuffing over the pork fillet and spread to within 4 cm (1½ inches) of the edge. Fold over the two short ends of the pork fillet, then roll up, Swiss-roll fashion, from a long side. Tie the roll with string at 4 cm (1½ inch) intervals.
5 Place the meat in a baking dish or casserole with a tight-fitting lid and add the orange juice. Cover and cook at 190°C (375°F) mark 5 for 45 minutes. Baste the meat with the cooking juices and cook for a further 10 minutes.
6 Transfer the meat to a warmed serving dish and keep warm. Pour the cooking juices into a saucepan, bring to the boil and cook until reduced by half. Strain, then stir in the remaining parsley.
7 Remove the string and serve the meat, cut into slices, with a little sauce poured over. Serve the remaining sauce separately.

Nutritional analysis	
285 kcals/1195 kJ	240 mcg Vitamin A ★ ★
31 g Protein	1.3 mg Vitamin B₁ ★ ★ ★ ★ ★
10 g Fat	21 mg Vitamin C ★ ★ ★ ★
20 g Carbohydrate	3.6 mg Zinc ★ ★
8.7 g Fibre ★ ★	

Sautéed Lambs' Kidneys

Combining kidneys, mushrooms and onions in a sherry sauce, this dish needs only the accompaniment of rice and a salad. Kidneys and liver are particularly rich in vitamins and minerals, such as vitamin B₁₂ and iron, both of which are vital for healthy red blood cells and the prevention of anaemia.

SERVES 4
16 baby onions, skinned
30 ml (2 tbsp) polyunsaturated oil
100 g (4 oz) button mushrooms
8 lambs' kidneys, skinned and cored
15 ml (1 tbsp) plain wholemeal flour
200 ml (7 fl oz) beef stock
15 ml (1 tsp) whole grain mustard
pepper
finely chopped fresh parsley, to garnish

1 Place the onions in a saucepan of boiling water and cook for 3–4 minutes. Drain.
2 Heat the oil in a saucepan and cook the onions and mushrooms over a high heat for 5 minutes or until the onions are browned.
3 Remove the onions and mushrooms from the pan with a slotted spoon and add the kidneys to the remaining oil. Cook quickly, stirring occasionally, for about 3 minutes or until the kidneys are browned. Remove from the pan.
4 Stir in the flour and cook for 1 minute. Remove from the heat and gradually stir in the stock and sherry, then bring to the boil and cook, stirring, until thick. Add the mustard and pepper.
5 Return the onions, mushrooms and kidneys to the sauce, reduce the heat, cover and simmer for 15–20 minutes or until the onions and kidneys are cooked. Serve garnished with chopped parsley.

Nutritional analysis	
215 kcals/895 kJ	20 mg Vitamin C ★ ★ ★
21 g Protein	62 mg Vitamin B$_{12}$ ★ ★ ★ ★ ★
11 g Fat	9.4 mg Iron ★ ★ ★
7.4 g Carbohydrate	2.9 mg Zinc ★ ★
2 g Fibre	

Liver with Satsumas

Liver is so rich in vitamins and minerals that one serving of this dish provides the recommended daily amount of iron and vitamin B$_{12}$. It also contains substantial amounts of folic acid. All three nutrients are vital for the production of red blood cells and therefore the supply of oxygen to all parts of the body, including the skin.

SERVES 4
2 satsumas or tangerines
450 g (1 lb) lamb's liver, sliced and cut lengthways into thin strips
30 ml (2 tbsp) plain wholemeal flour
pepper
30 ml (2 tbsp) polyunsaturated oil
1 onion, skinned and sliced
30 ml (2 tbsp) chopped fresh parsley

1 Using a sharp knife or vegetable peeler, pare the rind from the satsumas, then cut it into thin strips and set aside. Peel the satsumas and divide into segments. If using tangerines, remove the pips.
2 Toss the strips of liver in the flour and sprinkle with pepper to taste. Heat the oil in a non-stick frying pan, add the onion and cook for 5 minutes or until soft, stirring occasionally.
2 Add the liver and cook for about 5 minutes or until the liver changes colour, stirring occasionally.
4 Stir in the satsuma segments and parsley and cook for a further 2 minutes or until the fruit has softened slightly and the liver is tender. Serve hot, garnished with the strips of satsuma rind.

Nutritional analysis	
315 kcals/1315 kJ	467 mcg Vitamin A ★★
25 g Protein	264 mg Folic Acid ★★★★★
19 g Fat	35 mg Vitamin C ★★★★★
11 g Carbohydrate	95 mg Vitamin B$_{12}$ ★★★★★
2.4 g Fibre	12 mg Iron ★★★★★

Raspberry Chicken with Peaches

This attractive dish combines low-fat grilled chicken with the flavours of summer fruits. Raspberries contain useful amounts of iron, made more readily available by the presence also of vitamin C.

SERVES 4
4 chicken breast fillets, each weighing about 150 g (5 oz), skinned
250 g (9 oz) raspberries
30 ml (2 tbsp) lemon juice
30 ml (2 tbsp) clear honey
15 ml (1 tbsp) olive oil
30 ml (2 tbsp) red wine vinegar

15 ml (1 tbsp) reduced-sodium soy sauce, preferably naturally fermented shoyu
1 garlic clove, skinned and crushed
2.5 ml (½ tsp) mustard powder
salt and pepper
2 peaches, skinned, halved and stoned
sprigs of fresh herbs, to garnish

1 Make three slashes across the back and front of each chicken breast, but do not cut right through. Arrange in a shallow dish.
2 Reserve 25 g/l oz raspberries for serving and place the remainder in a blender or food processor with the lemon juice. Purée until smooth. Rub through a sieve and discard the seeds.
3 Add the honey, oil, vinegar, soy sauce, garlic, mustard powder and salt and pepper to taste to the raspberry sauce. Mix well and pour over the chicken breasts. Cover and leave to marinate for about 2 hours.
4 Drain the chicken, reserving the marinade, and place in the grill pan. Cook under a moderate grill for 20–25 minutes, turning frequently and basting with the marinade.
5 Brush the peach halves with marinade and arrange around the chicken breasts for the last 5 minutes of cooking.
6 To serve, arrange the chicken breasts on a warmed serving plate, spoon any sauce remaining in the grill pan over the chicken and garnish with fresh herbs. Fill the peach halves with the reserved raspberries and serve with the chicken.

Nutritional analysis	
280 kcals/1175 kJ	33 mg Vitamin C ★ ★ ★ ★ ★
35 g Protein	16 mg Niacin ★ ★ ★ ★
8.8 g Fat	0.86 mg Vitamin B$_6$ ★ ★
17 g Carbohydrate	2.5 mg Iron ★ ★
6.1 g Fibre ★ ★	

Honeyed Chicken

Shoyu is a naturally fermented Japanese soy sauce with a fuller flavour than chemically produced soy sauce. Look for the reduced-sodium variety. B complex vitamins necessary for energy production are present in this dish – B$_3$ (niacin), B$_6$ and pantothenic acid in particular. Niacin is essential for maintaining healthy skin and prevents pellagra – rough, scaly skin.

SERVES 4
2 garlic cloves, skinned and crushed
2.5 cm (1 inch) piece of fresh root ginger, peeled and finely chopped or 10 ml (2 tsp) ground ginger

30 ml (2 tbsp) reduced-sodium soy sauce, preferably naturally fermented shoyu
pinch of mustard powder
60 ml (4 tbsp) clear honey
4 chicken breasts, skinned

1 To make the marinade, mix together all the ingredients except the chicken. Rub the marinade well into both sides of the chicken pieces and leave to marinate for at least 1 hour, turning occasionally.
2 Place the chicken in a roasting tin with the marinade and cook at 190°C (375°F) mark 5 for 45 minutes–1 hour.

Nutritional analysis	
230 kcals/955 kJ	15 mg Niacin ★ ★ ★ ★
33 g Protein	0.79 mg Vitamin B$_6$ ★ ★
5 g Fat	525 mg Potassium ★
13 g Carbohydrate	1.3 mg Iron ★
0.1 g Fibre	

Chicken Parmigiana

Vitamin E enables blood vessels to open up and bring new supplies of blood to the skin. This dish is a good source of this vitamin.

SERVES 6

900 g (2 lb) aubergines, thickly sliced
polyunsaturated oil
700 g (1½ lb) chicken breast fillets, skinned
1 egg, beaten
50 g (2 oz) freshly grated Parmesan cheese
1 large onion, skinned and thinly sliced
1 garlic clove, skinned and crushed
400 g (14 oz) can chopped tomatoes
pinch of freshly grated nutmeg
5 ml (1 tsp) dried oregano
pinch of sugar
salt and pepper
175 g (6 oz) mozzarella cheese, sliced

1 Blanch the aubergine slices in boiling salted water for 2 minutes. Drain and refresh under cold water. Pat dry with absorbent kitchen paper. Brush each slice with a little oil and brown under a hot grill for a few minutes on each side. Leave to cool.
2 Dip the chicken fillets in the beaten egg and then in the Parmesan cheese. Cover and chill for 10–15 minutes.
3 Heat 15 ml (1 tbsp) oil in a frying pan and fry the onion with the garlic for about 5 minutes or until soft. Stir in the tomatoes, nutmeg, oregano and sugar. Add salt and pepper to taste. Spoon into a 2 litre (3½ pint) shallow ovenproof dish.
4 Heat a further 30 ml (2 tbsp) oil in the frying pan and quickly brown the chicken on both sides. Drain on absorbent kitchen paper.
5 Arrange overlapping rows of chicken, aubergine and mozzarella on top of the tomato mixture. Sprinkle with any remaining Parmesan cheese.
6 Bake in the oven at 190°C (375°F) mark 5 for 35–40 minutes or until the chicken is cooked and golden brown.

Nutritional analysis	
420 kcals/1745 kJ	178 mcg Vitamin A ★ ★
37 g Protein	23 mg Vitamin C ★ ★ ★ ★
26 g Fat	7.4 mcg Vitamin E ★ ★ ★ ★
9.3 g Carbohydrate	302 mg Calcium ★ ★ ★ ★
4.8 g Fibre ★	

Turkey and Ginger Stir-Fry

Quickly stir-frying these finely shredded pieces of vegetable and turkey uses less fat than other forms of frying. One of the functions of vitamin C is to protect vitamin E from destruction. Both vitamins are required to maintain healthy blood capillaries.

SERVES 4

30 ml (2 tbsp) polyunsaturated oil

4 spring onions, trimmed and roughly chopped

2.5 cm (1 inch) piece of fresh root ginger, peeled and cut into thin strips

1 garlic clove, skinned and crushed

450 g (1 lb) turkey breast fillets, skinned and cut into thin strips

1 red pepper, cored, seeded and sliced

1 green pepper, cored, seeded and cut into matchstick strips

1 leek, cut into thin strips

50 g (2 oz) shelled peanuts (with skins)

15 ml (1 tbsp) sesame seeds

15 ml (1 tbsp) reduced-sodium soy sauce, preferably naturally fermented shoyu

salt and pepper

1 Heat the oil in a large frying pan or wok. Add the spring onions, ginger and garlic and stir-fry for 1 minute.

2 Add the turkey and stir-fry for 3–4 minutes or until the turkey is evenly coloured. Add the pepper and leek and stir-fry for 2 minutes.

3 Add the peanuts, sesame seeds and soy sauce and continue stir-frying for a further 2–3 minutes or until the turkey is just tender. Add salt and pepper to taste. Serve piping hot with boiled rice.

Nutritional analysis	
305 kcals/1275 kJ	80 mg Vitamin C ★ ★ ★ ★ ★
30 g Protein	5.3 mcg Vitamin E ★ ★ ★
19 g Fat	2.5 mg Iron ★ ★
5.9 g Carbohydrate	2.8 mg Zinc ★ ★
2.6 g Fibre	

Chicken and Orange Kebabs

The combination of chicken livers, orange and watercress means this dish contains exceptional amounts of vitamin A – important for maintaining healthy mucous membranes and preventing infection.

SERVES 4
100 ml (4 fl oz) dry white wine
60 ml (4 tbsp) lemon juice
30 ml (2 tbsp) olive oil
1 garlic clove, skinned and crushed
15 ml (1 tbsp) chopped fresh tarragon
grated rind of 1 orange

pepper
450 g (1 lb) chicken breast fillets, skinned and cubed
225 g (8 oz) chicken livers, thawed if frozen, halved
TO GARNISH
2 oranges, peeled and segmented
watercress sprigs

1 Mix together the wine, lemon juice, oil, garlic, tarragon and orange rind. Add pepper to taste.
2 Pour the marinade over the chicken and livers, reserving about 75 ml (5 tbsp) for basting, and leave to marinate for at least 4 hours, turning several times.
3 Thread the chicken pieces and the livers evenly on to four long skewers and place under the grill.
4 Grill the kebabs for about 15 minutes, basting occasionally with the reserved marinade, and turning once during cooking. Serve hot, garnished with the orange segments and watercress.

Nutritional analysis	
320 kcals/1330 kJ	5262 mcg Vitamin A ★ ★ ★ ★ ★
36 g Protein	32 mg Vitamin B$_{12}$ ★ ★ ★ ★ ★
15 g Fat	58 mg Vitamin C ★ ★ ★ ★ ★
7 g Carbohydrate	6.4 mg Iron ★ ★ ★
1.5 g Fibre	2.9 mg Zinc ★ ★

Chicken and Avocado Stroganoff

Serve this unusual chicken dish with noodles and a mixed salad.
Niacin (vitamin B₃) and vitamin B₆ are two of the B complex vitamins
required for energy production within the body cells.

SERVES 4
500 g (1¼ lb) chicken breast
fillets, skinned
150 ml (¼ pint) dry white wine
1 avocado
15 ml (1 tbsp) French mustard
15 ml (1 tbsp) whole grain
mustard

150 g (5 oz) Greek-style natural
yogurt
15 ml (1 tbsp) snipped fresh
chives
salt and pepper

1 Arrange the chicken breasts in a single layer in a large frying
pan. Pour over the wine and 150 ml (¼ pint) water, cover and
simmer gently for 5–7 minutes or until the chicken is cooked.
2 Remove the chicken from the pan. Bring the cooking juices to a
rapid boil and boil, uncovered, for 5 minutes or until reduced by
half. Meanwhile, cut the chicken into strips. Peel and stone the
avocado and cut into strips.
3 Return the chicken to the pan with the French and whole grain
mustard and cook for 1–2 minutes, stirring constantly. Lower the
heat, then stir in the yogurt a spoonful at a time. Heat gently, then
add the avocado and snipped chives. Season to taste with salt and
pepper.

Nutritional analysis	
375 kcals/1575 kJ	14 mg Niacin ★ ★ ★ ★
35 g Protein	1 mg Vitamin B₆ ★ ★ ★
22 g Fat	10 mg Vitamin C ★ ★
3.7 g Carbohydrate	2.1 mg Iron ★
1.3 g Fibre	

Stir-Fried Duckling with Mange-Tout

Removing the skin from duck dramatically reduces the fat content;
duck flesh contains no more fat than chicken flesh.

SERVES 4

150 ml (¼ pint) chicken stock, skimmed

30 ml (2 tbsp) reduced-sodium soy sauce, preferably naturally fermented shoyu

15 ml (1 tbsp) cornflour

5 ml (1 tsp) light muscovado sugar

350 g (12 oz) duckling breast fillets, skinned

15 ml (1 tbsp) Hoisin sauce

15 ml (1 tbsp) dry sherry

30 ml (2 tbsp) polyunsaturated oil

1 garlic clove, skinned and crushed

2.5 cm (1 inch) piece of fresh root ginger, peeled and chopped

1 bunch of spring onions, trimmed and sliced into 2.5 cm (1 inch) lengths

230 g (8 oz) can whole water chestnuts, drained and thinly sliced

225 g (8 oz) mange-tout, topped and tailed

salt and pepper

1 Mix together the stock, soy sauce, half the cornflour and the sugar. Cut the duckling breasts into thin strips and mix with the remaining cornflour, Hoisin sauce and sherry.

2 Heat 15 ml (1 tbsp) oil in a wok or heavy-based frying pan and stir in the garlic and ginger. Cook gently for about 5 minutes or until soft, then turn up the heat. Add the duckling and stir-fry until the meat changes colour. Remove from the pan and set aside.

3 Heat the remaining oil in the pan and stir-fry the spring onions for 1 minute. Add the water chestnuts and mange-tout and cook for another minute.

4 Add the duckling and stock mixture and cook, stirring continually, until bubbling. Season to taste with salt and pepper and serve immediately.

Nutritional analysis	
280 kcals/1170 kJ	21 mg Vitamin C ★ ★ ★
22 g Protein	0.51 mg Vitamin B₁ ★ ★
12 g Fat	4.4 mg Iron ★ ★
21 g Carbohydrate	2.1 mg Zinc ★
3.5 g Fibre ★	

7

Vegetarian Main Dishes

Many people believe that a truly healthy diet can only be achieved if meat and fish are excluded altogether. Certainly, this would eliminate a large amount of saturated fat from the diet, and necessary protein and iron can be provided by other foods, such as pulses and grains. Even if you or your family are not vegetarian, a meat-free meal once or twice a week would certainly be of benefit. The main dishes here are based on fresh vegetables but many include dried pulses, rice or pasta to add nutrients or substance, while fresh herbs, nuts and cheese add flavour and texture.

Spicy Black Beans and Rice

Wash your hands immediately after preparing fresh chillies. The juices can irritate your skin especially of you touch your eyes or lips. The combination of beans (a pulse) and rice (a cereal) provides complete protein as good as animal protein.

SERVES 4

225 g (8 oz) black beans, soaked overnight and drained
30 ml (2 tbsp) olive oil
2 large onions, skinned and chopped
2.5 cm (1 inch) piece of fresh root ginger, peeled and grated
1 fresh green chilli, seeded and chopped
1 large green pepper, cored, seeded and chopped
1 large red pepper, cored, seeded and chopped
2 garlic cloves, skinned and crushed
10 ml (2 tsp) ground cumin
10 ml (2 tsp) ground coriander
5 tomatoes, roughly chopped
225 g (8 oz) canned tomatoes,
3 courgettes, trimmed and sliced
175 g (6 oz) brown rice
salt and pepper
1 large banana
5 ml (1 tsp) lemon juice
2 eggs, hard-boiled and chopped
parsley sprigs, to garnish

1 Place the beans in a large saucepan and cover with cold water. Bring to the boil and boil rapidly for 10 minutes, then lower the heat and simmer for 40–50 minutes or until tender.

2 Meanwhile, heat the oil in a large saucepan and cook the onions, ginger and chilli for 4–5 minutes or until the onions are soft. Add the peppers, garlic and spices and cook over a high heat for 1–2 minutes, stirring constantly.

3 Add the fresh and canned tomatoes with their juice. Bring to the boil and simmer for about 5 minutes or until reduced and thickened.

4 When the beans are cooked, drain and add to the vegetable mixture with the courgettes, rice and 450 ml (¾ pint) water. Bring to the boil, cover and simmer for 30 minutes or until the rice is tender. Season to taste with salt and pepper.

5 To serve, arrange the beans and rice on a large warmed serving dish. Peel and slice the banana and sprinkle with the lemon juice. Arrange on top with the hard-boiled eggs. Garnish with the parsley. Serve hot or cold.

Nutritional analysis	
530 kcals/2215 kJ	0.78 mg Vitamin B$_1$ ★ ★ ★ ★
24 g Protein	188 mg Folic Acid ★ ★ ★
14 g Fat	5.7 mcg Vitamin E ★ ★ ★
82 g Carbohydrate	11 mg Iron ★ ★ ★ ★ ★
23 g Fibre ★ ★ ★	225 mg Calcium ★ ★ ★
162 mg Vitamin C ★ ★ ★ ★ ★	

Lentil Roulade with Mushrooms

This dish is rich in calcium, providing more than half the recommended daily amount (RDA) for adults. During pregnancy and when breast feeding, women need more than twice as much calcium.

SERVES 4

175 g (6 oz) red lentils, rinsed
450 ml (¾ pint) vegetable stock
1 medium onion, skinned and sliced
568 ml (1 pint) semi-skimmed milk
bay leaves and slices of carrot and onion, to flavour
50 g (2 oz) polyunsaturated margarine

60 ml (4 tbsp) plain flour
1 bunch of watercress, rinsed
salt and pepper
freshly grated Parmesan cheese
3 eggs, separated
225 g (8 oz) button mushrooms
30 ml (2 tbsp) lemon juice

1 Put the lentils in a small saucepan and pour in the stock. Add the sliced onion and bring to the boil. Cover and simmer for about 20 minutes or until the lentils are soft and all the liquid has been absorbed. Stir occasionally to prevent the lentils sticking and boil to evaporate any remaining liquid at the end. Leave to cool slightly.

2 Meanwhile, bring the milk to the boil with the flavouring ingredients. Remove from the heat, cover and leave to infuse for about 20 minutes. Melt 25 g (1 oz) of the margarine in a small saucepan and stir in 30 ml (2 tbsp) of the flour followed by 200 ml (7 fl oz) strained, infused milk. Bring to the boil and cook for 1–2 minutes, stirring frequently.

3 In a blender or food processor, blend together the lentils, sauce, watercress and salt and pepper to taste. Blend until the lentils are almost smooth and the watercress finely chopped. Turn into a large bowl and leave until cold.

4 Meanwhile, grease and line the base of a 23 × 33 cm (9 × 13 inch) Swiss roll tin. Grease the paper and dust with Parmesan cheese.

5 Beat the egg yolks into the lentil mixture. Whisk the egg whites until stiff but not dry and fold into the lentil mixture. Spread in the tin.

6 Bake at 200°C (400°F) mark 6 for about 30 minutes or until well risen, golden brown and firm to the touch.

7 Meanwhile, slice the mushrooms. Cook quickly for 1-2 minutes in the remaining margarine. Stir in the remaining flour followed by the remaining strained milk. Bring to the boil and cook, stirring, for 1-2 minutes. Add the lemon juice and season to taste with salt and pepper. Keep warm over a low heat.

8 Have ready a large sheet of non-stick or greaseproof paper or foil sprinkled with Parmesan cheese. Flip the roulade over on to the paper and peel off the lining paper. Roll up immediately from the shortest end with the help of the sheet of paper. Lift on to a serving dish and serve straight away with the mushroom sauce.

Nutritional analysis	
450 kcals/1875 kJ	338 mcg Vitamin A ★ ★
26 g Protein	26 mg Vitamin C ★ ★ ★ ★ ★
20 g Fat	387 mg Calcium ★ ★ ★ ★
45 g Carbohydrate	5.7 mg Iron ★ ★ ★
8.4 g Fibre ★ ★	

Vegetable Risotto

Magnesium is a mineral which assists in many of the body's enzyme systems, such as energy production and maintaining the correct distribution of sodium, potassium and calcium between cell membranes.

SERVES 4
30 ml (2 tbsp) olive oil
50 g (2 oz) unsalted peanuts

50 g (2 oz) unsalted cashew nuts
25 g (1 oz) pine nuts

100 g (4 oz) brown rice
about 450 ml (¾ pint)
vegetable stock
4 celery sticks, trimmed and
cut into small pieces
2 courgettes, trimmed and
diced
1 yellow pepper, cored, seeded
and chopped

8 spring onions, trimmed and
cut diagonally into small
pieces
salt and pepper
30 ml (2 tbsp) chopped fresh
basil
2 eggs, hard-boiled and sliced
lemon wedges, to garnish

1 Heat the oil in a saucepan, add the nuts and rice and cook for 5 minutes or until the nuts are lightly toasted.
2 Pour in 450 ml (¾ pint) of the stock, then add the celery, courgettes, yellow pepper and spring onions. Season to taste with salt and pepper.
3 Bring to the boil, then reduce the heat and simmer gently for 30–40 minutes or until the rice is tender, stirring occasionally and adding more stock or a little water if necessary to prevent sticking.
4 Stir in the basil and mix well. Turn into a warmed serving dish. Top with the slices of hard-boiled egg and garnish with lemon wedges. Serve hot.

Nutritional analysis	
405 kcals/1695 kJ	0.5 mg Vitamin B$_6$ ★ ★
13 g Protein	4.2 mcg Vitamin E ★ ★ ★
28 g Fat	3 mg Iron ★ ★
29 g Carbohydrate	2.1 mg Zinc ★
5.5 g Fibre ★	118 mg Magnesium ★ ★
67 mg Vitamin C ★ ★ ★ ★ ★	

Vegetable Curry

The vitamins and minerals in vegetables are most concentrated just beneath the skin, so do not peel them. Potassium assists with protein synthesis within cells. Vitamin C is required to maintain collagen – a protein which forms connective tissue in the skin.

SERVES 4

15 ml (1 tbsp) polyunsaturated oil

1 onion, skinned and finely chopped

1 garlic clove, skinned and chopped

5 ml (1 tsp) coriander seeds, crushed

5 ml (1 tsp) ground turmeric

5 ml (1 tsp) ground cumin

2.5 ml (½ tsp) garam masala

300 ml (½ pint) vegetable stock

30 ml (2 tbsp) tomato purée

15 ml (1 tbsp) plain wholemeal flour

150 ml (¼ pint) low-fat natural yogurt

450 g (1 lb) courgettes, trimmed and thickly sliced

450 g (1 lb) carrots, scrubbed and cut into chunks

225 g (8 oz) potatoes, scrubbed and cut into chunks

1 parsnip, peeled and cut into chunks

450 g (1 lb) tomatoes, chopped

½ cauliflower, divided into florets

1 small red pepper, cored, seeded and cut into thin strips

15 ml (1 tbsp) chopped cashew nuts

salt and pepper

1 Heat the oil in a saucepan and cook the onion gently for 5 minutes or until soft. Add the garlic and spices and cook for 1 minute more. Add the stock and purée and bring to the boil. Lower the heat and simmer.

2 Blend the flour with the yogurt and stir into the spice mixture. Add the courgettes, carrots, potatoes and parsnip. Simmer for 5 minutes, then add the remaining vegetables and continue simmering for 15 minutes. Stir in the cashew nuts and season to taste with salt and pepper.

Nutritional analysis	
245 kcals/1030 kJ	786 mcg Vitamin A ★ ★ ★ ★ ★
11 g Protein	156 mg Folic Acid ★ ★ ★
6.9 g Fat	144 mg Vitamin C ★ ★ ★ ★ ★
38 g Carbohydrate	2001 mg Potassium ★ ★ ★ ★
11 g Fibre ★ ★	6.7 mg Iron ★ ★ ★

Coriander Noodles

This is a lovely quick dish to put together and can be varied to use whatever vegetables you have available. They are very lightly cooked so that none of their crunchy texture and little of their nutritive value is lost. The dish provides a good supply of vitamin B₁ (thiamin) and vitamin C. Both these water-soluble vitamins are easily lost during food preparation.

SERVES 2
2 ripe tomatoes, chopped
15 ml (1 tbsp) chopped fresh coriander
30 ml (2 tbsp) chopped fresh parsley
finely grated rind and juice of ½ lemon
30 ml (2 tbsp) olive oil
1 garlic clove, skinned and crushed
salt and pepper
100 g (4 oz) green beans, trimmed and halved
175 g (6 oz) courgettes, trimmed and sliced
225 g (8 oz) mixed green and white fresh tagliatelle
fresh herbs, to garnish

1 Mix the tomatoes with the coriander and parsley, lemon rind and juice, oil, garlic and salt and pepper to taste.
2 Steam the beans and courgettes for 5 minutes or until they are just cooked.
3 Meanwhile, cook the pasta in boiling salted water for about 8 minutes or until just tender. Drain well.
4 Place the tomato mixture in a saucepan and heat through gently. Add the steamed vegetables and mix them lightly together. Serve with the cooked tagliatelle and garnish with fresh herbs.

Nutritional analysis	
555 kcals/2325 kJ	404 mcg Vitamin A ★ ★ ★
17 g Protein	0.58 mg Vitamin B₁ ★ ★
17 g Fat	62 mg Vitamin C ★ ★ ★ ★ ★
88 g Carbohydrate	4.7 mg Iron ★ ★
12 g Fibre ★ ★	

Pasta Shells with Cheese and Walnuts

This is a very quick and easy pasta dish – ideal for a family supper. Among the nutrients it provides are calcium, phosphorus, iron and zinc, together with vitamin D. Both calcium and phosphorus, which form the structure of teeth, are dependent on vitamin D for absorption. There is very little chance of experiencing phosphorous deficiency because it is present in so many foods.

SERVES 4

275 g (10 oz) wholewheat pasta shells
25 g (1 oz) polyunsaturated margarine
225 g (8 oz) low-fat soft cheese
30 ml (2 tbsp) freshly grated Parmesan cheese
75 g (3 oz) walnuts, roughly chopped
salt and pepper

1 Cook the pasta in boiling salted water until just tender. Drain well.
2 In the same pan, melt the margarine, add the cheese and stir for 2–3 minutes or until heated through. Do not boil.
3 Add the Parmesan and walnuts, stir, then add the pasta. Mix well until evenly coated with sauce. Season to taste with salt and pepper. Serve immediately.

Nutritional analysis	
485 kcals/2025 kJ	155 mg Calcium ★ ★
22 g Protein	336 mg Phosphorus ★ ★ ★
21 g Fat	1.5 mg Iron ★
56 g Carbohydrate	1.8 mg Zinc ★
3 g Fibre ★	1.8 mcg Vitamin D ★

Gado Gado

This traditional Indonesian salad is made of a mixture of lightly cooked and raw vegetables which may be varied according to seasonal availability. It is served with a spicy sauce. Vitamin A (retinol) is provided in the form of carotene in the vegetables. This is converted to retinol by the body, so quantities of vitamin A are denoted 'retinol equivalents'.

SERVES 4

100 g (4 oz) French beans, trimmed
225 g (8 oz) white cabbage, finely shredded

100 g (4 oz) carrots, scrubbed
and cut into matchsticks
100 g (4 oz) fresh bean sprouts
5 cm (2 inch) piece of
cucumber, sliced
4 eggs, hard-boiled and sliced
50 g (2 oz) desiccated coconut
15 ml (1 tbsp) polyunsaturated
oil

1 small onion, skinned and
finely chopped
75 g (3 oz) natural crunchy
peanut butter
5 ml (1 tsp) hot chilli powder
5 ml (1 tsp) light muscovado
sugar
15 ml (1 tbsp) lime juice

1 Bring a saucepan of water to the boil, add the beans and cook
for 2 minutes. Add the cabbage and cook for a further 1 minute.
Drain, then run under cold water until completely cold. Drain
well.

2 Put the blanched vegetables in a large shallow bowl with the
carrots, and bean sprouts and mix well. Arrange the cucumber
and egg slices alternately over the vegetables. Chill while
preparing the sauce.

3 To make the peanut sauce, put the coconut in a bowl and pour
over 300 ml(½ pint) boiling water. Leave to infuse for 20 minutes,
then strain through a sieve over a bowl, using a wooden spoon to
press out as much liquid as possible. Reserve the liquid and discard
the coconut.

4 Heat the oil in a saucepan and cook the onion for about 5 minutes
or until softened. Add the peanut butter, chilli powder and sugar
and mix well. Stir in the strained coconut liquid and bring to the
boil. Simmer for 5 minutes or until the sauce has thickened.
Remove from the heat, stir in the lime juice and leave to cool. Serve
the salad with some of the sauce poured over and the remainder
served separately.

Nutritional analysis	
350kcals/1465 kJ	638 mcg Vitamin A ★ ★ ★ ★ ★
15 g Protein	36 mg Vitamin C ★ ★ ★ ★
28 g Fat	671 mg Potassium ★ ★
12 g Carbohydrate	103 mg Calcium ★ ★
8.1 g Fibre ★ ★	3.1 mg Iron ★ ★

Nut and Cheese Plait

This wholesome nut loaf is delicious served simply with its yogurt dressing and a mixed salad. The nuts, wholemeal bread and flour provide 25 per cent of the recommended daily amount of fibre. Western diets are notoriously low in fibre.

SERVES 6
175 g (6 oz) mixed nuts, eg.
almonds, brazil nuts, hazelnuts,
unsalted peanuts
175 g (6 oz) polyunsaturated
margarine
1 small onion, skinned and
chopped
10 ml (2 tsp) bottled green
peppercorns, drained and
chopped
cayenne

100 g (4 oz) fresh wholemeal
breadcrumbs
100 g (4 oz) Cheddar cheese,
grated
1 egg, beaten
salt and pepper
150 g (5 oz) plain white flour
150 g (5 oz) plain wholemeal
flour
150 ml (¼ pint) low-fat natural
yogurt
finely grated rind of 1 lemon

1 Roughly chop 100 g (4 oz) of the nuts and finely chop the remainder. Melt 25 g (1 oz) of the margarine in a frying pan, add the onion, peppercorns and 1.25 ml (¼ tsp) cayenne and cook for 2–3 minutes, stirring.
2 Remove from the heat and stir in the roughly chopped nuts, breadcrumbs and cheese with sufficient egg just to bind the ingredients together. (Reserve the remaining egg for glazing). Season to taste with salt and pepper, then leave to cool completely.
3 Meanwhile, place the flours and all but 15 ml (1 tbsp) finely chopped nuts in a bowl with a pinch of cayenne. Rub in the remaining margarine until the mixture resembles fine breadcrumbs. Stir in about 60 ml (4 tbsp) water and gradually bring the mixture together.
4 Roll out the pastry to a 25.5 × 33 cm (10 × 13 inch) rectangle. Using the rolling pin as support, carefully lift the pastry on to a baking sheet. Make 7.5 cm (3 inch) long slits at 2 cm (¾ inch) intervals along both long edges of the rectangle.
5 Spoon the filling down the centre of the pastry, leaving a 4 cm (1½ inch) border at the top and bottom. Brush the strips with beaten egg, then fold the top and bottom borders over. Work down the 'loaf', covering the filling with alternate strips of pastry to form a plaited effect. Leave to chill for 10 minutes.
6 Brush the loaf with egg and sprinkle over the remaining nuts. Bake at 200°C (400°F) mark 6 for about 35 minutes or until well browned.
7 Meanwhile, mix the yogurt with the lemon rind and a little

cayenne. Serve the loaf, warm and thickly sliced, accompanied by the yogurt dressing.

Nutritional analysis	
700 kcals/2930 kJ	363 mcg Vitamin A ★ ★ ★
20 g Protein	12 mcg Vitamin E ★ ★ ★ ★ ★
48 g Fat	327 mg Calcium ★ ★ ★
51 g Carbohydrate	3.6 mg Iron ★ ★
8.6 g Fibre ★ ★	3.5 mg Zinc ★ ★

Ratatouille Cheese Pie

The reduced-fat, high-fibre pastry covers a delicious Mediterranean-style filling.

SERVES 4
225 g (8 oz) plain wholemeal flour
1.25 ml (¼ tsp) salt
2.5 ml (½ tsp) easy-mix dried yeast
1 egg, size 3, beaten
30 ml (2 tbsp) polyunsaturated oil
1 onion, skinned and chopped
2 garlic cloves, skinned and crushed
1 aubergine, sliced
2 courgettes, trimmed and sliced
½ red pepper, cored, seeded and chopped
½ green pepper, cored, seeded and chopped
450 g (1 lb) tomatoes, chopped
2.5 ml (½ tsp) dried thyme
1.25 ml (¼ tsp) ground coriander
15 ml (1 tbsp) chopped fresh parsley
150 g (5 oz) Mozzarella cheese, diced
salt and pepper
sesame seeds, for sprinkling

1 Lightly grease a rectangular 20 × 25 cm (8 × 10 inch) ovenproof dish and set aside. To make the pastry, place the flour, salt and yeast in a bowl. Add a third of the beaten egg and 1.25 ml (¼ tsp) oil and mix well, adding about 100 ml (4 fl oz) tepid water to form a fairly soft dough. Knead lightly. Cover the bowl with a clean cloth and leave to rise in a warm place for 40 minutes.
2 Meanwhile, making the filling. Heat the remaining oil in a large saucepan and cook the onion for about 5 minutes or until soft. Add the garlic and cook for 1–2 minutes, then mix in the aubergine, courgettes, peppers and tomatoes. Add the thyme and coriander. Cover and cook over a moderate heat for 30 minutes, stirring occasionally.

3 Remove the lid, stir, then boil the mixture vigorously for 1–2 minutes to thicken. Pour into the ovenproof dish and mix in the parsley, cheese and salt and pepper to taste.

4 Knock back the dough and roll out thinly on a lightly floured surface. Use to cover the vegetable mixture and brush with half the remaining beaten egg. Bake at 200°C (400°F) mark 6 for 15 minutes.

5 Brush with the remaining egg and sprinkle with sesame seeds. Bake for a further 5 minutes. Serve hot.

Nutritional analysis	
430 kcals/1805kJ	304 mcg Vitamin A ★ ★
20 g Protein	77 mg Vitamin C ★ ★ ★ ★ ★
19 g Fat	6.5 mcg Vitamin E ★ ★ ★ ★
48 g Carbohydrate	277 mg Calcium ★ ★ ★
10 g Fibre ★ ★	

Stuffed Baked Aubergines

A good quantity of potassium is present in this dish. A high potassium intake is necessary for maintaining the water balance of body cells.

SERVES 4
2 aubergines
25 g (1 oz) polyunsaturated margarine
4 small tomatoes, skinned and chopped
15 ml (1 tbsp) chopped fresh marjoram
1 large onion, skinned and chopped
50 g (2 oz) fresh wholemeal breadcrumbs
salt and pepper
50 g (2 oz) cheese, grated
parsley sprigs, to garnish

1 Steam or boil the whole aubergines for about 30 minutes or until tender.

2 Cut the aubergines in half lengthways. Scoop out the flesh and chop finely. Reserve the aubergine shells.

3 Melt the margarine in a saucepan, add the tomatoes, marjoram and onion and cook gently for 10 minutes. Stir in the aubergine flesh and a few breadcrumbs. Season to taste with salt and pepper.

4 Stuff the aubergine shells with this mixture, sprinkle with the remaining breadcrumbs and then with the grated cheese. Place in a grill pan and grill until golden brown on top. Serve hot, garnished with parsley sprigs.

Nutritional analysis	
165 kcals/695 kJ	188 mcg Vitamin A ★ ★
6.5 g Protein	27 mg Vitamin C ★ ★ ★ ★ ★
9.7 g Fat	631 mg Potassium ★ ★
14 g Carbohydrate	158 mg Calcium ★ ★
6.5 g Fibre ★ ★	

Cauliflower and Courgette Bake

This makes an excellent lunch or supper dish which can be served simply with a mixed salad. Each portion contains plenty of vitamin C. One of this vitamin's many roles in the body is to help in the production of an anti-stress hormone.

SERVES 4
700 g (1½ lb) cauliflower
40 g (1½ oz) polyunsaturated margarine
225 g (8 oz) courgettes, trimmed and thinly sliced
45 ml (3 tbsp) plain wholemeal flour
150 ml (¼ pint) semi-skimmed milk
3 eggs, separated
salt and pepper
15 ml (1 tbsp) freshly grated Parmesan cheese

1 Divide the cauliflower into small florets, trimming off thick stalks and leaves. Cook in boiling salted water for 10 minutes or until just tender.
2 Meanwhile, in a separate pan, melt 15 g (½ oz) of the margarine, add the courgettes and cook for 5 minutes or until beginning to soften. Remove from the pan with a slotted spoon and drain on absorbent kitchen paper.
3 Melt the remaining margarine in the pan, stir in the flour and cook, stirring, for 1–2 minutes. Remove from the heat and gradually add the milk, whisking constantly. Bring to the boil, stirring, then lower the heat and simmer until thickened.
4 Drain the cauliflower well and place in a blender or food processor with the warm sauce, egg yolks and salt and pepper to taste. Blend together until evenly mixed, then turn into a large bowl.
5 Whisk the egg whites until stiff and carefully fold into the cauliflower mixture. Spoon half the mixture into a 1.6 litre (2¾ pint) soufflé dish. Arrange the courgettes on top, reserving a few for garnish, then cover with the remaining cauliflower mixture and reserved courgettes.

6 Sprinkle over the Parmesan cheese and bake in the oven at 190°C (375°F) mark 5 for 35–40 minutes or until golden. Serve immediately.

Nutritional analysis	
225 kcals/935 kJ	191 mcg Vitamin A ★ ★
12 g Protein	110 mg Vitamin C ★ ★ ★ ★ ★
14 g Fat	875 mg Potassium ★ ★
12 g Carbohydrate	133 mg Calcium ★ ★
5 g Fibre ★	2.5 mg Iron ★ ★

Vegetable Loaf with Tomato Sauce

Different types of dietary fibre are of different benefit to the body. One form of fibre, found in vegetables and fruit, is pectin. One of its functions is to lower blood cholesterol and fat levels.

SERVES 4
10 ml (2 tsp) polyunsaturated oil
350 g (12 oz) carrots, grated
350 g (12 oz) courgettes, trimmed and grated
225 g (8 oz) leeks, finely shredded
1 garlic clove, skinned and crushed
150 g (5 oz) fresh wholemeal breadcrumbs
75 g (3 oz) Cheddar cheese, grated
3 eggs, size 2, beaten
45 ml (3 tbsp) low-fat natural yogurt
30 ml (2 tbsp) chopped fresh parsley
salt and pepper
TOMATO SAUCE
1 kg (2¼ lb) ripe tomatoes, skinned and coarsely chopped
1 small onion, finely chopped
1 carrot, scrubbed and chopped
2 celery sticks, finely chopped
1 garlic clove, skinned and crushed
30 ml (2 tbsp) chopped fresh parsley
15 ml (1 tbsp) chopped fresh basil

1 Lightly grease a 900 g (2 lb) loaf tin and line the base with greased greaseproof paper. Heat the oil in a saucepan and gently cook the vegetables and garlic for 5 minutes. Drain off the liquid and mix the vegetables with the breadcrumbs, cheese, eggs, yogurt, parsley and salt and pepper to taste.
2 Transfer the mixture to the loaf tin and cover with greased

kitchen foil. Stand the tin in a roasting tin and add enough hot water to come halfway up the sides of the loaf tin. Bake at 180°C (350°F) mark 4 for 55–60 minutes or until set.

3 To make the sauce, put all the ingredients in a saucepan. Bring to the boil, cover and simmer for about 45 minutes or until the vegetables are soft. Purée the sauce in a blender or food processor, then reheat gently.

4 Ease the cooked loaf away from the tin with a palette knife and invert on to a warmed serving dish. Serve with the sauce.

Nutritional analysis	
350 kcals/1465 kJ	101 mg Vitamin C ★ ★ ★ ★ ★
20 g Protein	141 mg Folic Acid ★ ★ ★
15 g Fat	6.4 mcg Vitamin E ★ ★ ★ ★
37 g Carbohydrate	403 mg Calcium ★ ★ ★ ★ ★
14 g Fibre ★ ★ ★	6 mg Iron ★ ★ ★
1015 mcg Vitamin A ★ ★ ★ ★ ★	

8

Vegetable Accompaniments

Some main dishes need nothing more than lightly cooked fresh vegetables to accompany them, while others require something a little more elaborate. The vitamins found in vegetables are water-soluble, which means they can easily be lost in the cooking water if they are boiled. Steaming is therefore a healthier cooking method, retaining both flavour and a greater proportion of vitamins in the vegetables. Stir-frying is another alternative as the vegetables are cooked so lightly and quickly that fewer nutrients are lost. Similarly, vegetables cooked quickly in very little water in a microwave cooker contain more nutrients.

Celeriac with Tomato Sauce

The vegetables, wholemeal breadcrumbs and cheese supply potassium, a mineral involved in initiating peristalsis, the rhythmic movement of the gut muscle.

SERVES 4

15 ml (1 tbsp) olive oil
1 large onion, skinned and finely chopped
3 garlic cloves, skinned and crushed
350 g (12 oz) ripe tomatoes, skinned and finely chopped
15 ml (1 tbsp) tomato purée
30 ml (2 tbsp) red wine or red wine vinegar
60 ml (4 tbsp) chopped fresh parsley

5 ml (1 tsp) ground cinnamon
1 bay leaf
salt and pepper
2 heads of celeriac, total weight about 900 g (2 lb)
5 ml (1 tsp) lemon juice
50 g (2 oz) fresh wholemeal breadcrumbs
50 g (2 oz) freshly grated Parmesan cheese

1 To make the tomato sauce, heat the oil in a heavy-based saucepan and cook the onion and garlic gently for about 10 minutes or until very soft and lightly coloured.

2 Add the tomatoes, tomato purée, wine, parsley, cinnamon, bay leaf and salt and pepper to taste. Add 450 ml (¾ pint) hot water and bring to the boil, stirring with a wooden spoon to break up the tomatoes. Lower the heat, cover and simmer for 30 minutes, stirring occasionally.

3 Meanwhile, peel the celeriac, then cut into chunky pieces, dropping each piece immediately into a bowl of water to which the lemon juice has been added, to prevent discoloration.

4 Drain the celeriac, then plunge quickly into a large pan of boiling salted water. Return to the boil and blanch for 10 minutes.

5 Drain the celeriac well, then put in an ovenproof dish. Pour over the tomato sauce (discarding the bay leaf), then sprinkle the breadcrumbs and cheese evenly over the top.

6 Bake the celeriac in the oven at 190°C (375°F) mark 5 for 30 minutes or until the celeriac is tender when pierced with a skewer and the topping is golden brown. Serve hot, straight from the dish.

Nutritional analysis	
180 kcals/750 kJ	57 mg Vitamin C ★ ★ ★ ★ ★
11 g Protein	1333 mg Potassium ★ ★ ★
8 g Fat	334 mg Calcium ★ ★ ★ ★
16 g Carbohydrate	4.3 mg Iron ★ ★
13 g Fibre ★ ★ ★	

Sautéed Courgettes with Chives

Vitamins C and E mutually protect each other from destruction. Vitamin C is present in the courgettes, herbs and lemon juice, while polyunsaturated oils and margarine provide vitamin E.

SERVES 4
15 g (½ oz) polyunsaturated margarine
15 ml (1 tbsp) polyunsaturated oil
450 g (1 lb) courgettes, trimmed and thinly sliced

grated rind and juice of ½ lemon
salt and pepper
15 ml (1 tbsp) snipped fresh chives

1 Heat the margarine and oil in a saucepan and cook the courgettes over a moderate heat, uncovered, for 5–8 minutes or until tender but still slightly crisp. Add the lemon rind and juice and season to taste with salt and pepper.
2 Turn the courgettes into a heated serving dish, sprinkle fresh chives over them and serve immediately, while still hot.

Nutritional analysis	
80 kcals/345 kJ	72 mcg Vitamin A
1.4 g Protein	12 mg Vitamin C ★ ★
7 g Fat	2.8 mcg Vitamin E ★ ★
3.8 g Carbohydrate	291 mg Potassium
0.6 g Fibre	

Spinach with Raisins and Nuts

Like all dark green leafy vegetables, spinach contributes not only folic acid, but plenty of minerals, particularly iron. Even though spinach is also a source of oxalic acid which binds some of the iron, making it unobtainable, considerable amounts of iron are still available, aided by the presence of vitamin C.

SERVES 4
900 g (2 lb) spinach, trimmed and rinsed
25 g (1 oz) raisins, rinsed
10 ml (2 tsp) olive oil
25 g (1 oz) hazelnuts, coarsely chopped

1 garlic clove, skinned and crushed
15 ml (1 tbsp) lemon juice
salt and pepper
lemon wedges, to garnish

1 Put the spinach in a large saucepan with just the water that clings to its leaves. Heat rapidly until the spinach sizzles, then lower the heat, add the raisins and cook for 4 minutes, stirring occasionally.

2 Meanwhile, heat the oil in a heavy-based frying pan and cook the nuts and garlic over a low heat until the nuts are lightly toasted.

3 Drain any water from the spinach and add the spinach to the frying pan. Cook, stirring, over a very low heat for 3–4 minutes. Stir in the lemon juice and season to taste with salt and pepper. Serve immediately with a wedge of lemon for each person.

Nutritional analysis	
125 kcals/525 kJ	25 mg Iron ★ ★ ★ ★
5.3 g Protein	81 mg Vitamin C ★ ★ ★ ★ ★
6.3 g Fat	0.53 mg Vitamin B$_6$ ★ ★
13 g Carbohydrate	282 mg Folic Acid ★ ★ ★ ★
3.2 g Fibre ★	

Roasted Oatmeal Vegetables

Carrots are renowned for their carotene content. As vitamin A, carotene helps to maintain healthy mucous membranes lining such areas as the intestine and bronchial tubes, thus preventing disease-producing organisms from entering the body.

SERVES 6
450 g (1 lb) medium onions, skinned
450 g (1 lb) carrots, scrubbed and cut into large chunks
450 g (1 lb) parsnips, peeled and cut into large chunks

75 ml (5 tbsp) polyunsaturated oil
175 g (6 oz) coarse oatmeal
5 ml (1 tsp) paprika
salt and pepper

1 Cut the onions into quarters, keeping the root end intact.

2 Put the carrots and parsnips in a saucepan of water, bring to the boil and cook for 2 minutes. Drain well.

3 Heat 30 ml (2 tbsp) of the oil in the saucepan and replace the carrots and parsnips. Add the onions, oatmeal and paprika and season to taste with salt and pepper. Stir gently to coat the vegetables.

4 Put the remaining oil in a large roasting tin and heat in the oven at 200°C (400°F) mark 6. When very hot, add the vegetables and oatmeal mixture and baste.

5 Roast in the oven for about 1 hour or until the vegetables are just tender and golden brown. Baste occasionally during cooking. Spoon into a warmed serving dish and sprinkle over any oatmeal 'crumbs'. Serve hot.

Nutritional analysis	
305 kcals/1265 kJ	1500 mcg Vitamin A ★ ★ ★ ★ ★
6.1 g Protein	23 mg Vitamin C ★ ★ ★ ★
15 g Fat	7.5 mcg Vitamin E ★ ★ ★ ★
38 g Carbohydrate	117 mg Calcium ★ ★ ★
8.2 g Fibre ★ ★	

Potato and Garlic Purée

Beat the chives into the potato just before serving, otherwise they'll discolour. Potatoes are the greatest source of vitamin C in the Western diet – not because they are a concentrated source of the vitamin but because they are eaten in such large quantities.

SERVES 4
700 g (1½ lb) old potatoes, peeled and cut into chunks
2 garlic cloves, skinned and chopped
salt and pepper

150 ml (¼ pint) semi-skimmed milk, warmed
15 g (½ oz) polyunsaturated margarine
snipped fresh chives

1 Put the potatoes and garlic in a saucepan and cover with water, adding a little salt. Bring to the boil, cover and simmer for 20 minutes or until the potatoes are tender.

2 Drain the potatoes, then return them to the pan, cover and place over a low heat to dry them a little. Mash the potatoes, adding the milk and margarine. Season to taste with salt and pepper and, just before serving, add the chives. Sprinkle more snipped chives over the surface.

Nutritional analysis	
180 kcals/755 kJ	23 mg Vitamin C ★ ★ ★ ★
4.6 g Protein	0.19 mg Vitamin B$_1$ ★
3.9 g Fat	929 mg Potassium ★ ★
34 g Carbohydrate	65 mg Calcium ★
3.3 g Fibre ★	

Brussels Sprouts with Hazelnuts

Green leafy vegetables, including Brussels sprouts, are a valuable source of folic acid – a B vitamin essential for healthy red blood cells as well as the construction of the nervous system in the developing unborn child.

SERVES 6
900 g (2 lb) Brussels sprouts,
trimmed
25 g (1 oz) hazelnuts
40 g (1½ oz) polyunsaturated
margarine

1 garlic clove, skinned and
crushed
salt and pepper

1 Cook the sprouts in boiling salted water for about 10 minutes or until just tender.
2 Meanwhile, toast the hazelnuts. Cool slightly, then rub off their skins and roughly chop.
3 Drain the sprouts, melt the margarine in the saucepan, add the garlic and cook for 1 minute. Stir in the sprouts and reheat gently. Season to taste with salt and pepper and sprinkle the chopped nuts over to serve.

Nutritional analysis	
105 kcals/440 kJ	160 mcg Vitamin A ★ ★
6.4 g Protein	135 mg Vitamin C ★ ★ ★ ★ ★
6.9 g Fat	168 mg Folic Acid ★ ★ ★
4.7 g Carbohydrate	4 mcg Vitamin E ★ ★
6.6 g Fibre ★ ★	

Steamed Greens with Mushrooms

Steaming the spring greens retains both their vitamins and their crunchiness. Vitamin C is destroyed in alkaline conditions – therefore, bicarbonate of soda should never be added to vegetable dishes to retain their vibrant green colour.

SERVES 4

225 g (8 oz) spring greens (stalks discarded), finely shredded

100 g (4 oz) mushrooms, sliced
juice of 1 lime or ½ lemon
salt and pepper
15 ml (1 tbsp) sunflower seeds

1 Place the spring greens in a steamer over a saucepan of gently boiling water and steam for 6–8 minutes or until almost cooked but still crunchy.
2 Meanwhile, put the mushrooms, lime juice and 30 ml (2 tbsp) water in a large saucepan and cook for 3 minutes. Drain off all but 15 ml (1 tbsp) of the liquid, then add the spring greens to the pan. Season to taste with salt and pepper and cook over a high heat for 2 minutes.
3 Place in a warmed serving dish, scatter the sunflower seeds over and serve hot.

Nutritional analysis	
30 kcals/120 kJ	375 mcg Vitamin A ★ ★ ★
2.1 g Protein	19 mg Vitamin C ★ ★ ★ ★
1.4 g Fat	68 mg Folic Acid ★ ★
2.2 g Carbohydrate	1.2 mg Iron ★
2.9 g Fibre	

Stir-Fried Green Beans with Mustard Seeds

Dark brown patches of skin, such as occur during pregnancy or while taking the contraceptive pill, have been attributed to folic acid deficiency.

SERVES 4
15 ml (1 tbsp) polyunsaturated oil
15 ml (1 tbsp) black mustard seeds
2 garlic cloves, skinned and finely chopped
5 ml (1 tsp) seeded and crushed dried red chillies

450 g (1 lb) green beans, cut into 2.5 cm (1 inch) pieces
1 small onion, skinned and finely chopped
15 ml (1 tbsp) lemon juice
salt and pepper

1 Heat the oil in a heavy-based saucepan or wok and cook the mustard seeds, stirring, until the seeds start sizzling and begin to turn brown. Add the garlic and chillies and continue cooking, stirring, until the garlic begins to colour.
2 Add the beans and onion and continue cooking, stirring, for about 5 minutes or until the beans are tender but still crisp. Add the lemon juice and cook for about 30 seconds longer. Season to taste with salt and pepper and serve at once.

Nutritional analysis	
90 kcals/385 kJ	27 mg Vitamin C ★ ★ ★ ★ ★
4.1 g Protein	2.1 mcg Vitamin E ★ ★
5.3 g Fat	71 mg Folic Acid ★ ★
7.7 g Carbohydrate	1.6 mg Iron ★
3.8 g Fibre ★	

Stir-Fried Asparagus

The lightly toasted sesame seeds sprinkled over the asparagus give a nutty flavour to this deliciously simple dish. The sesame seeds and corn oil contain essential fatty acids that help transport vitamin A into the body from the intestinal tract.

SERVES 4

25 ml (1½ tbsp) sesame seeds
450 g (1 lb) fresh asparagus
15 ml (1 tbsp) polyunsaturated oil
6 spring onions, trimmed and finely chopped
pepper
5 ml (1 tsp) freshly grated horseradish

1 Put the sesame seeds on a baking sheet and lightly toast at 200°C (400°F) mark 6 for 8–10 minutes. Set aside.

2 Discard the woody ends of the asparagus spears and scrape the stalks to remove any coarse scales. Cut the asparagus diagonally into 2.5 cm (1 inch) pieces.

3 Heat the oil in a frying pan or wok and cook the asparagus and spring onions for 1 minute, stirring. Season to taste with pepper and horseradish and sprinkle in the sesame seeds. Cook briskly for a further 1–2 minutes. Do not overcook the asparagus; it should be very crunchy. Serve hot or cold.

Nutritional analysis	
80 kcals/340 kJ	9.2 mg Vitamin C ★ ★
2.1 g Protein	2.4 mcg Vitamin E ★ ★
7.2 g Fat	86 mg Calcium ★
2.8 g Carbohydrate	1.3 mg Iron ★
1.1 g Fibre	

9

Seasonal Salads

In recent years, salads have become more and more imaginative, using a wide range of ingredients and tossed in exciting dressings. Salads may now be made of crisply cooked vegetables, pasta, rice, grains or pulses, and may include fruit, cheese, nuts, seeds and herbs of all sorts. They can be served all year round, using vegetables such as cabbage instead of lettuce, and apples instead of tomatoes to make crunchy combinations such as the winter salad on page 184. There are main dish salads here as well as those to serve as an accompaniment. Since they are made up of fresh, mostly raw or lightly cooked ingredients, they are all full of goodness and will add valuable nutrients to any diet.

Red Cabbage with Pears

Good quantities of folic acid and vitamin C are present in this dish. Vitamin C is required by folic acid to convert it into its active form within the body.

SERVES 6 AS AN
ACCOMPANIMENT
900 g (2lb) red cabbage
450 g (1 lb) firm pears
15 g (½ oz) polyunsaturated
margarine

1 garlic clove, skinned and
crushed
salt and pepper
150 ml (¼ pint) chicken stock
30 ml (2tbsp) lemon juice

1 Finely shred the cabbage. Peel, quarter, core and thickly slice the pears.
2 Mix together the margarine and garlic and use to grease the sides of a 3.4 litre (6 pint) casserole. Spoon half the cabbage into the dish, followed by a layer of pears. Season to taste with salt and pepper. Repeat the layers, ending with the pears.
3 Pour over the stock and lemon juice, cover the dish tightly and bake at 170°C (325°F) mark 3 for about 2 hours or until the cabbage is just tender. Adjust the seasoning and stir before serving.

Nutritional analysis	
75 kcals/305 kJ	87 mg Vitamin C ★ ★ ★ ★ ★
2.9 g Protein	141 mg Folic Acid ★ ★ ★
2.1 g Fat	533 mg Potassium ★
11 g Carbohydrate	85 mg Calcium ★
6.4 g Fibre ★ ★	

Crunchy Winter Salad

Fresh fruit and vegetables provide plenty of vitamin C in this tasty salad, and the calcium is provided by the yogurt and cheese. Both these nutrients are needed for strong bone and tooth formation.

SERVES 4 AS A MAIN COURSE
2 dessert apples
finely grated rind and juice of
½ lemon

45 ml (3 tbsp) polyunsaturated
oil
150 ml (¼ pint) low-fat natural
yogurt

salt and pepper
225 g (8 oz) red cabbage,
trimmed and finely sliced
1 small onion, skinned and finely
sliced
2 celery sticks, trimmed and
sliced

100 g (4 oz) Cheddar cheese,
diced
100 g (4 oz) shelled unsalted
peanuts
celery leaves, to garnish

1 Quarter and core the apples, then cut into chunks. Toss in 30 ml (2 tbsp) lemon juice.
2 To make the dressing, whisk the remaining lemon juice with the grated rind, oil, yogurt and salt and pepper to taste.
3 Put the cabbage, onion, celery, apple, cheese and peanuts in a large salad bowl, pour over the dressing and toss well. Adjust the seasoning, garnish with celery leaves and serve with warm wholemeal rolls.

Nutritional analysis	
410 kcals/1705 kJ	38 mg Vitamin C ★ ★ ★ ★ ★
16 g Protein	8 mcg Vitamin E ★ ★ ★ ★
32 g Fat	336 mg Calcium ★ ★ ★
14 g Carbohydrate	2.3 mg Zinc ★
5.8 g Fibre ★	

Tomato Salad with Fennel

Recent studies suggest that high intakes of carotene (which is a precursor of vitamin A) help reduce the skin's sensitivity to ultraviolet light, thus protecting it from the damaging rays of strong sunlight.

SERVES 4 AS AN
ACCOMPANIMENT
15 g (½ oz) sunflower seeds
450 g (1 lb) tomatoes, sliced

¼ bulb Florence fennel, finely
chopped
30 ml (2 tbsp) olive oil
salt and pepper

1 Place the sunflower seeds in a small heavy-based frying pan. Heat gently until pale golden brown, turning frequently so the seeds do not burn. Set aside to cool.

2 Arrange the tomatoes and fennel in a shallow bowl. Spoon over the oil and season to taste with salt and pepper. Mix gently until well coated. Add the sunflower seeds and toss gently. Serve at once.

Nutritional analysis	
105 kcals/440 kJ	113 mcg Vitamin A ★
1.8 g Protein	43 mg Folic Acid ★
8.7 g Fat	23 mg Vitamin C ★ ★ ★ ★
5.1 g Carbohydrate	397 mg Potassium ★
2 g Fibre	

Celeriac Salad

Mayonnaise is very high in fat so using half mayonnaise, half yogurt not only reduces the fat content but also makes a delicious dressing.

*SERVES 4 AS AN
ACCOMPANIMENT*
450 g (1 lb) celeriac, scrubbed
10 ml (2 tsp) lemon juice
60 ml (4 tbsp) mayonnaise
*60 ml (4 tbsp) low-fat natural
yogurt*
10 ml (2 tsp) Dijon mustard
salt and pepper

*15 ml (1 tbsp) capers, well
drained and finely chopped*
*15 ml (1 tbsp) very finely
chopped gherkin*
*15 ml (1 tbsp) finely chopped
fresh tarragon*
5 ml (1 tsp) anchovy essence
*chopped fresh parsley, to
garnish*

1 Peel the celeriac and cut into matchstick strips, dropping each piece immediately into a bowl of water to which the lemon juice has been added, to prevent discoloration.
2 To make the dressing, mix the mayonnaise with the yogurt and mustard in a salad bowl. Season to taste with salt and pepper.
3 Drain the celeriac and mix into the dressing with the capers, gherkin, tarragon and anchovy essence. Garnish with chopped parsley before serving.

Nutritional analysis	
145 kcals/605 kJ	9.2 mg Vitamin C ★ ★
5.1 g Protein	503 mg Potassium ★
12 g Fat	108 mg Calcium ★ ★
4.6 g Carbohydrate	1.9 mg Iron ★
4.8 g Fibre ★	

Chicken and Grape Salad

*This subtly-flavoured light salad is perfect for a summer lunch.
Serve with fresh French bread or a rice salad. The B vitamins
riboflavin, niacin and B_6 are all present in notable quantities. They
all play a role in energy production within the body.*

SERVES 4 AS A MAIN COURSE   90 ml (6 tbsp) lemon juice
1.4 kg (3 lb) chicken   45 ml (3 tbsp) clear honey
1 medium onion, skinned   150 ml (¼ pint) soured cream
1 carrot, peeled   225 g (8 oz) green grapes
1 bay leaf   50 g (2 oz) raisins
6 peppercorns   salt and pepper
2 eggs   lettuce, to serve

1 Put the chicken in a large saucepan with the onion, carrot, bay
leaf and peppercorns. Pour in enough water just to cover and
poach for about 1 hour or until tender. Cool for at least 2 hours in
the stock, then remove and cut the flesh into bite-sized pieces,
discarding skin and bones.
2 Beat the eggs with 60 ml (4 tbsp) lemon juice and the honey. Put
in the top of a double saucepan or in a basin standing over a
saucepan of hot water and cook, stirring, until thick. Remove from
the heat, cover with damp greaseproof paper and leave to cool for
45 minutes.
3 Fold the cream into the cold egg and lemon mixture.
4 Halve the grapes, remove the seeds and add the grapes to the
chicken with the remaining lemon juice, the raisins and the sauce.
Season to taste with salt and pepper.
5 Pile the salad into a lettuce-lined serving dish. Serve at room
temperature.

Nutritional analysis	
480 kcals/2005 kJ	0.68 mg Vitamin B₆ ★ ★
45 g Protein	9.6 mg Niacin ★ ★ ★
21 g Fat	18 mg Vitamin C ★ ★ ★
29 g Carbohydrate	423 mcg Vitamin A ★ ★ ★
2.2 g Fibre	3.4 mg Zinc ★ ★

Grape, Watercress and Stilton Salad

The fat-soluble vitamins A and E present in this dish are very important for healthy skin. Vitamin E not only protects vitamin A from destruction but also helps to generate new skin.

SERVES 4 AS AN
ACCOMPANIMENT
45 ml (3 tbsp) polyunsaturated
oil
15 ml (1 tbsp) lemon juice
5 ml (1 tsp) poppy seeds

pinch of light muscovado sugar
salt and pepper
175 g (6 oz) Stilton cheese
225 g (8 oz) black grapes
1 bunch of watercress

1 In a jug, whisk together the oil, lemon juice, poppy seeds, sugar and salt and pepper to taste.
2 Cut the rind off the Stilton and cut the cheese into 2 cm (¾ inch) cubes. Toss well in the prepared dressing until completely coated. Cover and chill in the refrigerator for 1 hour.
3 Meanwhile, halve the grapes and remove the pips. Place in a bowl, cover and chill in the refrigerator.
4 Trim the watercress of any tough root ends. Wash thoroughly, drain and pat dry.
5 To serve, toss together the grapes, watercress, Stilton and dressing in a salad bowl. Serve immediately.

Nutritional analysis	
350 kcals/1455 kJ	266 mcg Vitamin A ★ ★
12 g Protein	14 mg Vitamin C ★ ★ ★
29 g Fat	6.1 mcg Vitamin E ★ ★ ★ ★
9.4 g Carbohydrate	217 mg Calcium ★ ★ ★
0.9 g Fibre	

Pepper Salad

Peppers and parsley are concentrated sources of vitamin C and one portion of this dish supplies in the region of 166 milligrams. Body saturation of this vitamin occurs between 100 and 150 milligrams with any excess being excreted. Removing the skins from the peppers makes them more digestible.

SERVES 4 AS AN
ACCOMPANIMENT
2 red peppers
1 green pepper
1 yellow pepper
15 ml (1 tbsp) white wine
vinegar
30 ml (2 tbsp) polyunsaturated
oil

5 ml (1 tsp) clear honey
15 ml (1 tbsp) chopped fresh
parsley
pepper
10 ml (2 tsp) sesame seeds,
toasted

1 Place the peppers under a hot grill and cook for 10–15 minutes, turning frequently, until the skins are shrivelled and partially blackened.
2 Peel the peppers under cold running water and then cut in half and discard the cores and seeds. Cut the peppers into 2.5 cm (1 inch) pieces and place in a salad bowl.
3 Put the vinegar, oil, honey and parsley in a screw-topped jar, add pepper to taste and shake vigorously until well blended.
4 Pour over the peppers and sprinkle with the toasted sesame seeds just before serving.

Nutritional analysis	
80 kcals/325 kJ	97 mcg Vitamin A ★
2.1 g Protein	166 mg Vitamin C ★ ★ ★ ★ ★
5.8 g Fat	3.2 mcg Vitamin E ★ ★
5.1 g Carbohydrate	1.4 mg Iron ★
1.9 g Fibre	

Courgette and Pepper Salad

Salad dressings usually contribute large amounts of fat to the diet in the form of oil. The dressing used here substitutes tomato purée for the oil, making the overall dish practically fat-less.

SERVES 4 AS AN
ACCOMPANIMENT
60 ml (4 tbsp) cider vinegar
30 ml (2 tbsp) tomato purée
5 ml (1 tsp) dark muscovado
sugar
1.25 ml (¼ tsp) chilli powder
1.25 ml (¼ tsp) mustard powder
1 small garlic clove, skinned and
crushed

2.5 ml (½ tsp) paprika
225 g (8 oz) courgettes,
trimmed and thinly sliced
½ yellow pepper, cored,
seeded and cut into thin strips
½ red pepper, cored, seeded
and cut into thin strips
100 g (4 oz) button mushrooms,
thinly sliced

1 Put the vinegar, tomato purée, sugar, chilli powder, mustard, garlic and paprika into a bowl and mix well.
2 Add the courgettes, strips of pepper and sliced mushrooms and toss together lightly. Leave to stand for 30 minutes before serving to let the flavours develop.

Nutritional analysis	
35 kcals/140 kJ	80 mcg Vitamin A ★
2.2 g Protein	54 mg Vitamin C ★ ★ ★ ★
0.5 g Fat	484 mg Potassium ★
5.3 g Carbohydrate	1.2 mg Iron ★
1.3 g Fibre	

Curried Apple Coleslaw

Spices, such as curry powder, coriander and cinnamon, are concentrated sources of minerals, including potassium, calcium and iron. Here, the spices are combined in a creamy dressing to pour over a crisp salad.

SERVES 4 AS AN
ACCOMPANIMENT
10 ml (2 tsp) mild curry powder
5 ml (1 tsp) ground coriander

2.5 ml (½ tsp) ground cinnamon
45 ml (3 tbsp) mayonnaise
45 ml (3 tbsp) low-fat natural
yogurt

15 ml (1 tbsp) lemon juice
salt and pepper
½ medium white cabbage, finely
shredded
4 celery sticks, chopped
2 red eating apples, cored and
thinly sliced

8 radishes, trimmed and sliced
1 bunch of spring onions,
trimmed and chopped
10 ml (2 tsp) caraway seeds

1 To make the dressing, mix together the curry powder, coriander, cinnamon, mayonnaise, yogurt and lemon juice. Season to taste with salt and pepper.
2 Place the salad ingredients in a bowl and pour the dressing over. Toss gently, then sprinkle with the caraway seeds. Serve at once.

Nutritional analysis	
165 kcals/695 kJ	54 mg Vitamin C ★ ★ ★ ★ ★
4.5 g Protein	713 mg Potassium ★ ★
10 g Fat	201 mg Calcium ★ ★ ★
16 g Carbohydrate	5.6 mg Iron ★ ★ ★
6.2 g Fibre ★ ★	

Oriental Salad

Reduced-sodium shoyu, available from healthfood shops, contains one-third less salt than ordinary soy sauces. Using the low-sodium alternative does not compromise its contribution to the flavour of any dish. Excessive salt intake, by people susceptible to hypertension, leads to fluid retention and puffy skin. Serve this oriental salad in pitta bread pockets to accompany barbecued food.

SERVES 8 AS AN
ACCOMPANIMENT
1 large cucumber
1 small head Chinese leaves
1 red pepper
100 g (4 oz) button mushrooms
225 g (8 oz) bean sprouts
30 ml (2 tbsp) reduced-sodium
soy sauce, preferably naturally
fermented shoyu

15 ml (1 tbsp) peanut butter
30 ml (2 tbsp) sesame oil
30 ml (2 tbsp) rice or wine
vinegar
pepper
50 g (2 oz) shelled unsalted
peanuts

1 Cut the cucumber in half lengthways and scoop out the seeds. Cut the halves into 5 cm (2 inch) sticks, leaving the skin on.
2 Shred the Chinese leaves, wash and drain well. Cut the red pepper in half and remove the core and seeds. Cut the flesh into thin strips. Wipe and slice the mushrooms. Rinse the bean sprouts and drain well.
3 Just before serving, put the soy sauce in a large bowl and mix in the peanut butter, oil, vinegar and pepper to taste. Add the salad ingredients and the peanuts and toss well together.

Nutritional analysis	
110 kcals/465 kJ	39 mg Vitamin C ★ ★ ★ ★
4.6 g Protein	0.18 mg Vitamin B$_1$ ★
8.2 g Fat	1.2 mcg Vitamin E ★
4.9 g Carbohydrate	1.7 mg Iron ★
2.5 g Fibre	

Golden Salad

The carotene content of this dish is particularly high. Found in yellow fruit and dark green vegetables, it imparts the 'golden' colour to this dish.

SERVES 4 AS AN
ACCOMPANIMENT
½ pineapple, about 700 g
(1½ lb), with the leafy crown
attached
3 carrots, scrubbed and grated

50 g (2 oz) dried stoned dates,
rinsed and finely chopped
75 ml (3 fl oz) unsweetened
orange juice
50 g (2 oz) flaked almonds,
toasted

1 Completely cut out the pineapple flesh, without damaging the skin. Cut out and discard the core and cut the pineapple flesh into bite-sized pieces over a small bowl to catch the juices. Reserve the pineapple juice and the shell.
2 Place the pineapple pieces, carrots and dates in a bowl. Pour over the reserved pineapple juice and the orange juice and toss well. Put the salad into the pineapple shell, scatter the almonds on top and serve.

Nutritional analysis	
165 kcals/680 kJ	1062 mcg Vitamin A ★ ★ ★ ★ ★
3.3 g Protein	36 mg Vitamin C ★ ★ ★ ★ ★
6.7 g Fat	2.8 mcg Vitamin E ★ ★
24 g Carbohydrate	1.5 mg Iron ★
5.5 g Fibre ★	

Hedgerow Salad

Plenty of raw salads in the diet, where minimal destruction of vital vitamins occurs, contribute hugely to healthy skin. If you don't grow them in your garden, healthfood shops and some large supermarkets sell edible flowers.

SERVES 4 AS AN
ACCOMPANIMENT
1 small bunch of dandelion
leaves
a few chicory leaves
1 small curly endive
50 g (2 oz) sorrel
a few edible flowers such as
primulas or nasturtiums

50 g (2 oz) walnuts, chopped
30 ml (2 tbsp) walnut oil
60 ml (4 tbsp) lemon juice
1 garlic clove, skinned and
crushed
salt and pepper

1 Break all the leaves into bite-sized pieces and place in a large bowl. Sprinkle over the flowers.
2 Mix together the remaining ingredients and pour over the salad. Toss and serve immediately.

Nutritional analysis	
145 kcals/605 kJ	212 mcg Vitamin A ★ ★
2.3 g Protein	17 mg Vitamin C ★ ★ ★
14 g Fat	2.9 mcg Vitamin E ★ ★
2.3 g Carbohydrate	97 mg Folic Acid ★ ★
1.5 g Fibre	2.5 mg Iron ★ ★

Cauliflower, Banana and Date Salad

*Large amounts of vitamin C and valuable amounts of folic acid are
contributed by this dish. Folic acid is as important as iron for the
production of red blood cells.*

SERVES 4 AS AN
ACCOMPANIMENT
1 small red pepper, cored and
seeded
½ small cauliflower, divided
into florets
1 large banana, peeled and
sliced
75 g (3 oz) fresh or dried
dates, rinsed, stoned and
halved

40 g (1½ oz) blue cheese, such
as Stilton or Roquefort
60 ml (4 tbsp) mayonnaise
30 ml (2 tbsp) low-fat natural
yogurt
½ small endive, trimmed
a few parsley sprigs, to
garnish

1 Cut the pepper into short sticks and mix with the cauliflower,
banana and dates.
2 Mash the cheese until smooth, then gradually stir in the mayonnaise and yogurt. Pour over the salad ingredients and mix together
until well coated.
3 Arrange the endive leaves on a serving platter and place the
prepared salad on top. Garnish with the parsley sprigs.

Nutritional analysis	
220 kcals/920 kJ	143 mcg Vitamin A ★
5.7 g Protein	78 mg Vitamin C ★ ★ ★ ★
16 g Fat	92 mg Folic Acid ★ ★
14 g Carbohydrate	0.35 mg Vitamin B$_6$ ★
3.5 g Fibre ★	1.5 mg Iron ★

Sprouted Salad

Sprouting your own pulses and seeds is great fun, ensuring a wonderful source of vitamin C, particularly in the winter months. If you don't have the time to sprout your own, mung or aduki beans, alfalfa and chick-peas can all be bought ready sprouted at healthfood shops and some of the larger supermarkets.

SERVES 4 AS AN
ACCOMPANIMENT
50 g (2 oz) alfalfa seeds
50 g (2 oz) mung or aduki beans
50 g (2 oz) chick-peas
1 punnet of mustard and cress
½ red pepper, cored, seeded and diced
2 tomatoes, sliced

30 ml (2 tbsp) tahini
45 ml (3 tbsp) low-fat natural yogurt
1 garlic clove, skinned and crushed (optional)
15–30 ml (1–2 tbsp) lemon juice
1.25 ml (¼ tsp) ground cumin
pepper

1 Before sprouting, check all pulses for broken beans or pods which will not sprout, and discard.
2 If using a bought sprouter, follow the instructions given. Otherwise, soak the pulses for 10–15 hours to enable germination to start. Rinse well.
3 To sprout the pulses, put them in a glass jar with a piece of muslin held with a rubber band over the top to enable you to pour in and drain out water. Keep the sprouting pulses in a warm dark place, rinsing twice a day. Alfalfa will take 5–6 days to sprout, mung or aduki beans will take 3–6 days and chick-peas 2–3 days. Place in daylight just before the sprouts have reached their full length.
4 Rinse and drain the sprouts well, then mix with the remaining salad ingredients in a bowl. Stir the tahini, yogurt, garlic (if using), lemon juice and cumin together, adding a little more yogurt if the dressing is too thick. Season to taste with pepper. Pour over the salad and toss just before serving.

Nutritional analysis	
160 kcals/675 kJ	31 mg Vitamin C ★ ★ ★ ★ ★
11 g Protein	70 mg Folic Acid ★ ★
5.1 g Fat	155 mg Calcium ★ ★
19 g Carbohydrate	5.2 mg Iron ★ ★ ★
8.7 g Fibre ★ ★	1.4 mg Zinc ★

Bean, Cheese and Avocado Salad

*The hummus and yogurt mixture is a low-fat alternative to using oil
in the dressing for this salad. It also increases the calcium content
of the dish. Serve as a main course with hot wholemeal rolls or
baked jacket potatoes.*

SERVES 4 AS A MAIN COURSE
225 g (8 oz) dried red kidney
beans, soaked in cold water
overnight
60 ml (4 tbsp) hummus
60 ml (4 tbsp) low-fat natural
yogurt
finely grated rind and juice of
½ lemon
1.25 ml (¼ tsp) Tabasco sauce
salt and pepper

175 g (6 oz) Edam cheese,
rinded and diced
1 small onion, skinned and
finely chopped
2 celery sticks, trimmed and
finely chopped
2 tomatoes, skinned and
chopped
1 ripe avocado
celery leaves, to garnish

1 Drain the kidney beans and rinse under cold running water. Put
in a saucepan, cover with fresh cold water and bring to the boil.
Boil rapidly for 10 minutes, then simmer for 1–1½ hours or until
tender.
2 Drain the beans, rinse with cold water and drain again. Place
the beans in a salad bowl. Mix together the hummus, yogurt, lemon
rind and juice, Tabasco and salt and pepper to taste. Pour over the
beans and toss together, then leave until cold.
3 Add the cheese, onion, celery and tomatoes to the beans and toss
again to mix the ingredients together. Cover and chill in the refrigerator until ready to serve.
4 Just before serving, peel the avocado, cut in half and remove the
stone. Chop the flesh into chunky pieces. Fold the avocado pieces
gently into the bean salad and check the seasoning. Garnish with
celery leaves and serve.

Nutritional analysis	
465 kcals/1954 kJ	5.4 mg Iron ★ ★ ★
28.3 g Protein	3.7 mg Zinc ★ ★ ★
26.3 g Fat	150 mcg Vitamin A ★ ★
31.3 g Carbohydrate	138 mg Folic Acid ★
16.5 g Fibre ★ ★ ★	22.6 mg Vitamin C ★ ★ ★ ★
471 mg Calcium ★ ★ ★ ★ ★	2.75 mcg Vitamin E ★ ★

Mixed Grain and Nut Salad

The protein in peanuts combines with that in grains to make 'complete proteins' – as valuable as animal protein which the body can use for growth and repair. High in vitamins A, C and E, this dish provides zinc as well. All are essential for wound healing.

SERVES 4 AS A MAIN COURSE
75 g (3 oz) whole wheat grains
75 g (3 oz) brown rice
75 g (3 oz) bulgar wheat
100 g (4 oz) frozen sweetcorn kernels
25 g (1 oz) unskinned almonds, chopped
25 g (1 oz) unskinned hazelnuts
50 g (2 oz) natural roasted peanuts
90 ml (6 tbsp) polyunsaturated oil
45 ml (3 tbsp) cider or wine vinegar
15 ml (1 tbsp) whole grain mustard
1 garlic clove, skinned and crushed

a few crushed cardamom seeds
salt and pepper
1 small green pepper, cored, seeded and diced
1 small red pepper, cored, seeded and diced
1 carrot, scrubbed and grated
1 celery stick, trimmed and finely sliced
50 g (2 oz) button mushrooms, finely sliced
60 ml (4 tbsp) snipped fresh chives
60 ml (4 tbsp) chopped fresh parsley
60 ml (4 tbsp) bean sprouts

1 Rinse and cook the whole wheat grains in boiling water for 1½ hours or until tender. Drain and set aside to cool.
2 Meanwhile, cook the brown rice in boiling water for 30 minutes or until tender. Drain and cool.
3 Put the bulgar wheat in a saucepan, add 175 ml (6 fl oz) water and bring to the boil. Cover and simmer for 10 minutes or until the water is absorbed. Set aside to cool.
4 Cook the sweetcorn kernels in boiling salted water for 5–8 minutes. Drain and rinse under cold water. Chill until required.
5 Place the nuts in a single layer on a shallow pan and toast them under a medium grill until they begin to colour.

6 To make the dressing, put the oil, vinegar, mustard, garlic, cardamom seeds and salt and pepper to taste into a screw-topped jar and shake until thoroughly mixed. Just before serving, mix all the grains, vegetables, herbs and nuts together in a bowl. Pour the dressing over the salad, mix lightly and serve.

Nutritional analysis	
595 kcals/2485 kJ	94 mg Vitamin C ★ ★ ★ ★
14 g Protein	17 mcg Vitamin E ★ ★ ★ ★ ★
37 g Fat	146 mg Calcium ★ ★
55 g Carbohydrate	5.1 mg Iron ★ ★ ★
9.8 g Fibre ★ ★	3 mg Zinc ★ ★
555 mcg Vitamin A ★ ★	

10
Barbecue Dishes

A barbecue is popular for informal summer entertaining and it is also a healthy method of cooking since, as when grilling, fat from meat or poultry can drip away. The recipes included here are those that can also be eaten easily in a bun or in pitta bread pockets and can be served with salads. For a change from burgers and kebabs, however, try some of the delicious fish dishes included. To end the meal, you will find the Barbecued Bananas (page 207), cooked in orange juice and cinnamon, impossible to resist.

Marinated Lamb Kebabs

The mineral, zinc, is often lost during food preparation. These lamb kebabs provide plenty for the many enzyme functions carried out by the body.

SERVES 4
150 ml (¼ pint) low-fat natural yogurt
2.5 cm (1 inch) piece of fresh root ginger, peeled and grated
2 garlic cloves, skinned and crushed
30 ml (2 tbsp) chopped fresh mint
10 ml (2 tsp) crushed cumin seeds

5 ml (1 tsp) ground turmeric
5 ml (1 tsp) salt
2.5 ml (½ tsp) chilli powder
700 g (1½ lb) lean boned shoulder of lamb, trimmed of excess fat and cut into cubes
2 medium onions
mint sprigs and lemon wedges, to garnish

1 Put the yogurt in a large bowl and add the ginger, garlic, mint, cumin, turmeric, salt and chilli powder. Stir well to mix.
2 Add the cubes of lamb to the bowl and stir to coat in the marinade. Cover and refrigerate for 1–2 days, turning occasionally.
3 When ready to cook, skin the onions and cut into quarters with a sharp knife.
4 Thread the lamb and onion quarters alternately on to eight oiled kebab skewers, pressing the pieces as close together as possible. Reserve any leftover marinade.
5 Barbecue or grill the kebabs for about 10 minutes or until the lamb is browned on the outside and pink in the centre. Turn frequently and brush with the reserved marinade. Serve hot, garnished with mint sprigs and lemon wedges.

Nutritional analysis	
340 kcals/1420 kJ	24 mg Vitamin C ★ ★ ★ ★
40 g Protein	0.31 mg Vitamin B₁ ★ ★ ★
16 g Fat	152 mg Calcium ★ ★
9.2 g Carbohydrate	6.1 mg Iron ★ ★ ★
2.6 g Fibre	7.4 mg Zinc ★ ★ ★ ★

Greek-Style Kebabs

Lamb is a good source of potassium, iron and zinc. Zinc is essential for the action of the enzymes needed to release carbon dioxide from the blood into the lungs for expiration from the body.

SERVES 4
14 stoned black olives
350 g (12 oz) lean minced leg
of lamb
1 garlic clove, skinned and
crushed
1 onion, skinned and finely
chopped
75 g (3 oz) fresh brown
breadcrumbs
25 ml (1½ tbsp) tomato purée
15 ml (1 tbsp) sesame seeds

2.5 ml (½ tsp) ground mixed
spice
pepper
8 shallots or small onions,
skinned
1 red pepper, cored, seeded
and cubed
30 ml (2 tbsp) olive oil
45 ml (3 tbsp) lemon juice
30 ml (2 tbsp) chopped fresh
coriander

1 Finely chop six of the olives and put in a mixing bowl with the lamb, garlic, onion, breadcrumbs, tomato purée, sesame seeds and mixed spice. Season to taste with pepper and mix together well. Form into twelve small sausage-shapes and chill for 30 minutes.

2 Thread four kebab skewers with the lamb rolls, shallots, pepper and remaining olives. Blend the oil, lemon juice and coriander together and brush over the kebabs.

3 Barbecue or grill for 8–10 minutes or until cooked, turning and brushing occasionally with the coriander mixture.

Nutritional analysis	
320 kcals/1330 kJ	136 mcg Vitamin A ★ ★
22 g Protein	68 mg Vitamin C ★ ★ ★ ★
20 g Fat	108 mg Calcium ★ ★
14 g Carbohydrate	3.9 mg Iron ★ ★
4.3 g Fibre ★	4.5 mg Zinc ★ ★

Hamburgers

Lean minced beef is essential for healthy hamburgers. Ideally, mince chuck steak yourself or buy the best mince available.

MAKES 4
450 g (1 lb) lean minced beef
100 g (4 oz) fresh wholemeal
breadcrumbs
1 small onion, skinned and
grated

2 carrots, scrubbed and grated
30 ml (2 tbsp) chopped fresh
mixed herbs
1 egg, beaten
salt and pepper

1 Mix together all the ingredients and divide into four. With lightly floured hands, shape into four thick, round burgers.
2 Barbecue or grill for 15 minutes or until cooked to taste, turning once during cooking. Serve in wholemeal buns with lettuce and chutney.

Nutritional analysis Per Burger	
220 kcals/930 kJ	357 mcg Vitamin A ★ ★ ★
27 g Protein	14 mg Vitamin C ★ ★ ★
7.4 g Fat	4 mg Iron ★ ★
12 g Carbohydrate	5.7 mg Zinc ★ ★ ★
3.4 g Fibre ★	

Hake Steaks in Lime

Hake is from the same family as cod, and although it is similar in shape it has closer-textured white flesh. It is available fresh from June to January and widely available frozen throughout the rest of the year.

SERVES 4
grated rind and juice of 4 limes
30 ml (2 tbsp) chopped fresh
basil
75 ml (3 fl oz) dry white wine
2 garlic cloves, skinned and
crushed

5 ml (1 tsp) paprika
15 ml (1 tbsp) olive oil
salt and pepper
4 hake or cod steaks, each
weighing about 175 g (6 oz)
lime slices and fresh basil
leaves, to garnish

1 Mix together the lime rind and juice, basil, wine, garlic, paprika and oil, with salt and pepper to taste, in a large bowl. Add the hake steaks and leave to marinate for 2 hours, carefully turning the fish at least once.

2 Remove the steaks from the marinade and barbecue or grill for about 8 minutes on each side, basting with the marinade, until cooked through and the flesh flakes easily. Discard any remaining marinade. Serve immediately, garnished with lime slices and basil leaves.

Nutritional analysis	
170 kcals/720 kJ	0.7 g Fibre
28 g Protein	17 mg Vitamin C ★ ★ ★
4.9 g Fat	618 mg Potassium ★ ★
1.6 g Carbohydrate	

Monkfish and Mussel Brochettes

Molluscs, like shellfish, are high in minerals, such as iron. One serving of this dish provides over half the recommended daily intake of iron.

SERVES 6
900 g (2 lb) monkfish, skinned and boned
36 cooked mussels
12 lean bacon rashers, rinded and halved
25 g (1 oz) polyunsaturated margarine, melted
60 ml (4 tbsp) chopped fresh parsley
finely grated rind and juice of 1 lime or lemon
3 garlic cloves, skinned and crushed
pepper
shredded lettuce, bay leaves, and lime or lemon wedges, to serve

1 Cut the fish into cubes. Using a sharp knife, shell the mussels. Reserve the mussels and discard the shells.

2 Roll the bacon rashers up neatly. Thread the cubed fish, mussels and bacon alternately on to six oiled kebab skewers.

3 Mix together the margarine, parsley, lime rind and juice, garlic and pepper to taste.

4 Place the brochettes on an oiled grill or barbecue rack. Brush with the margarine mixture, then barbecue or grill for 15 minutes. Turn the brochettes frequently during cooking and brush with the margarine mixture with each turn.

5 Arrange the hot brochettes on a serving platter lined with shredded lettuce. Garnish with bay leaves and lime wedges.

Nutritional analysis	
245 kcals/1030 kJ	18 mg Vitamin C ★ ★ ★
39 g Protein	649 mg Potassium ★ ★
9.1 g Fat	171 mg Calcium ★ ★
1 g Carbohydrate	6.4 mg Iron ★ ★ ★
1.1 g Fibre	2.4 mg Zinc ★ ★
171 mcg Vitamin A ★ ★	

Mustard Chicken Drumsticks

It is important that chicken is cooked through thoroughly to destroy any micro-organisms that may be present in the meat. If frozen chicken is used, it should be thawed completely before cooking.

SERVES 4
25 g (1 oz) polyunsaturated margarine
45 ml (3 tbsp) whole grain mustard
grated rind and juice of 1 lemon
10 ml (2 tsp) chopped fresh rosemary
salt and pepper
8 chicken drumsticks
rosemary sprigs, to garnish

1 In a bowl, cream the margarine until soft. Work in the mustard a little at a time using a wooden spoon. Grate in the lemon rind, then gradually beat in 15 ml (1 tbsp) lemon juice, the chopped rosemary and salt and pepper to taste.

2 Spread the mustard mixture over the chicken drumsticks, coating evenly. Chill in the refrigerator if not cooking immediately.

3 Barbecue or grill the drumsticks for 10–15 minutes on each side or until the skin is crisp and golden and the chicken is tender. Serve garnished with rosemary.

Nutritional analysis	
260 kcals/1080 kJ	16 mg Vitamin C ★ ★ ★
33 g Protein	464 mg Potassium ★
13 g Fat	53 mg Calcium ★
2 g Carbohydrate	1.7 mg Iron ★
1 g Fibre	2.2 mg Zinc ★

Barbecued Red Mullet

Red mullet is a good source of the B vitamins B_3 (niacin), B_6 and B_{12}. Vitamins B_3 and B_6 are required for energy production, while B_{12} is required for red blood cell production. B_{12} deficiency can result in pernicious anaemia.

SERVES 4
4 red mullet, cleaned
2 lemons
pepper
fresh herb sprigs

15 ml (1 tbsp) polyunsaturated oil
lemon wedges and fresh herb sprigs, to garnish

1 Remove the scales from the fish by scraping from tail to head with the back of a knife. Rinse well.
2 Slice one of the lemons. Sprinkle pepper inside each fish and stuff with fresh herbs and lemon slices. Squeeze over the juice from the remaining lemon.
3 Barbecue or grill for 10–15 minutes, turning carefully once and brushing with the oil. Serve garnished with herbs and lemon wedges.

Nutritional analysis	
300 kcals/1245 kJ	35 mg Vitamin C ★ ★ ★ ★ ★
43 g Protein	11 mg Niacin ★ ★ ★ ★
12 g Fat	0.98 mg Vitamin B_6 ★ ★ ★
1.5 g Carbohydrate	2.2 mg Vitamin B_{12} ★ ★ ★ ★
2.1 g Fibre	2.4 mg Iron ★ ★

Tandoori Chicken

Skinning the chicken dramatically reduces the fat content of this popular Indian-style dish. Fat contributes twice as much energy, gram for gram, as protein or carbohydrate. Plenty of B vitamins are also present to assist in energy production from the above nutrients.

SERVES 4
4 chicken quarters, skinned
30 ml (2 tbsp) lemon juice
1 garlic clove, skinned
2.5 cm (1 inch) piece of fresh
root ginger, peeled and chopped
1 green chilli, seeded
60 ml (4 tbsp) low-fat natural
yogurt

5 ml (1 tsp) ground cumin
5 ml (1 tsp) garam masala
15 ml (1 tbsp) paprika
5 ml (1 tsp) salt
lemon wedges and onion rings,
to serve

1 Using a sharp knife or skewer, prick the flesh of the chicken pieces all over. Put in an ovenproof dish and rub the lemon juice into the chicken flesh. Cover and leave for 30 minutes.
2 Meanwhile, put the garlic, ginger, chilli and 15 ml (1 tbsp) water in a blender or food processor and blend to a smooth paste.
3 Add the yogurt, cumin, garam masala, paprika and salt and mix together. Pour over the chicken so that it is completely covered. Cover and leave to marinate at room temperature for 5 hours. Turn once or twice during this time.
4 Barbecue or grill the chicken for 20–25 minutes or until tender, basting with the marinade and turning occasionally. Serve with lemon wedges and onion rings.

Nutritional analysis	
330 kcals/1380 kJ	0.29 mg Vitamin B_1 ★ ★
53 g Protein	0.48 mg Vitamin B_2 ★ ★ ★ ★ ★
11 g Fat	20 mg Niacin ★ ★ ★
3.6 g Carbohydrate	1.1 mg Vitamin B_6 ★ ★
1.7 g Fibre	5.7 mg Iron ★ ★ ★

Barbecued Bananas

Bananas are a good source of vitamin B_6. Deficiency of this vitamin may lead to an unbalanced facial skin often referred to as a 'combination' skin.

SERVES 4
4 large bananas
25 g (1 oz) demerara sugar
grated rind and juice of 1 large
orange
grated rind and juice of 1 lime
2.5 ml (½ tsp) ground
cinnamon

25 g (1 oz) polyunsaturated
margarine
orange and lime slices, to
decorate
thick natural yogurt, to serve

1 Cut four large rectangles of kitchen foil. Peel the bananas, then place one on each piece of foil. Prick them in several places with a fine skewer.
2 Mix together the sugar, orange rind and juice, lime rind and juice and cinnamon. Pour slowly over the bananas, dividing it equally between them. Dot with the margarine.
3 Bring the two long sides of the foil up over one banana, then fold the join over several times to seal thoroughly.
4 Fold up the ends of the foil so that the banana is enclosed completely and the juices cannot run out during cooking. Repeat with the remaining three bananas.
5 Place the parcels on the barbecue or grill and cook for 15 minutes, turning them once during cooking.
6 To serve, open the parcels carefully and transfer the bananas to individual serving dishes. Pour over the juices which have collected in the foil and decorate with orange and lime slices. Serve with thick natural yogurt.

Nutritional analysis	
200 kcals/835 kJ	26 mg Vitamin C ★ ★ ★ ★ ★
1.7 g Protein	0.61 mg Vitamin B_6 ★ ★
5.5 g Fat	1.8 mcg Vitamin E ★
39 g Carbohydrate	484 mg Potassium ★
4.3 g Fibre ★	

Vegetable Kebabs

It is best to leave the cutting of vegetables until the last minute to reduce vitamin C loss. Losses occur as a result of exposure to air, light and heat, thus making less available to the body. Vary your selection of vegetables, using those in season.

SERVES 4
8 button onions, skinned
12 button mushrooms
½ red pepper, cored, seeded and cubed
½ green pepper, cored, seeded and cubed
½ yellow pepper, cored, seeded and cubed
1 courgette, trimmed and cut into 8 chunks

8 firm cherry tomatoes
8 bay leaves
5 ml (1 tsp) whole grain mustard
45 ml (3 tbsp) unsweetened pineapple juice
15 ml (1 tbsp) olive oil
pepper

1 Thread the prepared vegetables and bay leaves on to four kebab skewers. Combine the mustard, pineapple juice, oil and pepper to taste in a small bowl. Brush the kebabs with this mixture.
2 Barbecue or grill the kebabs for 6–8 minutes, turning frequently and brushing with the remaining pineapple mixture. Serve hot.

Nutritional analysis	
75 kcals/305 kJ	32 mg Folic Acid ★
2.3 g Protein	108 mg Vitamin C ★ ★ ★ ★
4.6 g Fat	1.3 mcg Vitamin E ★
6.1 g Carbohydrate	520 mg Potassium ★
2.4 g Fibre	

11
Puddings and Desserts

Based on delicious fresh or dried fruits, there are desserts here to suit every occasion. Choose a fruit salad or sorbet to end a rich and filling meal, or something more substantial if the main course has been a light fish, chicken or vegetable dish. The recipes have been chosen for their low sugar content. Some do use muscovado sugar, which is less refined than white sugar, while others use honey as a sweetener. Avoid serving cream or custard with puddings or desserts; low-fat natural yogurt is a far healthier alternative.

Exotic Fruit Salad

All these tropical fruits should be available at large supermarkets. You can add or substitute others, either fresh or canned in natural juices. Papaya contains enzymes which are used to tenderize meat. It is also believed they assist with the digestion of protein.

SERVES 4
900 g (2 lb) ripe pineapple
1 mango or small papaya
1 guava or banana, sliced

1 passion fruit or pomegranate
4 lychees or rambutans
1 kiwi fruit

1 Cut the pineapple in half lengthways, with the leaves attached. Remove the core in a wedge from each half and discard. Cut the flesh away from the skin, cut it into small chunks and place in a bowl. Scrape out any remaining flesh and juice with a spoon and add to the bowl.
2 Peel the mango or papaya and remove the stone or seeds. Cut the flesh into cubes and add to the pineapple with the guava or banana.
3 Cut the passion fruit or pomegranate in half and scoop out the seeds with a teaspoon. Add the seeds to the pineapple.
4 Peel the lychees or rambutans and cut in half. Remove and discard the stones and add to the bowl of fruit.
5 Peel the kiwi fruit and cut the flesh into round slices. Add to the bowl of fruit and stir.
6 Spoon the fruit salad into the pineapple halves. Cover and chill until required.

Nutritional analysis	
130 kcals/545 kJ	183 mcg Vitamin A ★ ★
1.5 g Protein	0.13 mg Vitamin B$_1$ ★
0.3 g Fat	141 mg Vitamin C ★ ★ ★ ★ ★
32 g Carbohydrate	592 mg Potassium ★
4.2 g Fibre ★	

Pears with Blackcurrant Sauce

Blackcurrants are renowned for their vitamin C content. Ensuring good Vitamin C intake when you have a cold reduces the severity of the symptoms.

SERVES 4
4 cooking pears, peeled, but with stalks left intact
225 g (8 oz) frozen blackcurrants

50 g (2 oz) light muscovado sugar

1 Place the pears, blackcurrants, sugar and 100 ml (4 fl oz) water in a saucepan and bring slowly to the boil.
2 Lower the heat, cover and simmer for about 25 minutes, turning once, until the pears are soft but not mushy. Gently remove the pears and place them on individual plates.
3 Increase the heat and boil the blackcurrants rapidly for 3–4 minutes or until the liquid has reduced slightly. Press through a fine sieve and pour a little sauce over each pear. Serve at once or chill.

Nutritional analysis	
115 kcals/490 kJ	116 mg Vitamin C ★ ★ ★ ★ ★
0.9 g Protein	388 mg Potassium ★
0 g Fat	51 mg Calcium ★
30 g Carbohydrate	1 mg Iron
8 g Fibre ★ ★	

Fruit Jelly

Prunes and oranges are traditionally eaten for their laxative qualities. This is due to their high fibre and potassium content.

SERVES 4
225 g (8 oz) no-soak prunes
thinly pared rind of 1 orange
150 ml (¼ pint) unsweetened orange juice

15 g (½ oz) powdered gelatine
3 large oranges, peeled and segmented

1 Put the prunes, orange rind and 450 ml (¾ pint) water in a saucepan. Cook gently for 10–15 minutes or until the prunes are tender. Drain, reserving the cooking liquid, and discard the rind. Halve the prunes and remove the stones.

2 Add the orange juice and enough cold water to the prune liquid to make it up to 600 ml (1 pint).

3 Sprinkle the gelatine over 45 ml (3 tbsp) cold water in a heatproof bowl and leave to soften for 1 minute. Place over a saucepan of gently simmering water and stir until the gelatine has dissolved. Leave to cool, then mix into the fruit juices.

4 Place a 1.1 litre (2 pint) jelly mould or dish in a large mixing bowl containing ice cubes. Pour a little of the jelly mixture into the mould to a depth of 2.5 cm (1 inch) and allow to set.

5 Arrange either a layer of halved prunes or orange segments on top of the jelly. Cover with a little jelly and allow to set. Add more jelly, then more fruit, allowing each layer to set before starting the next. Continue until all the jelly and fruit have been used. Chill for 3 hours or until set.

Nutritional analysis	
155 kcals/655 kJ	99 mg Vitamin C ★ ★ ★ ★
5.8 g Protein	74 mg Folic Acid ★ ★
0 g Fat	788 mg Potassium ★ ★
36 g Carbohydrate	2.1 mg Iron ★
11 g Fibre ★ ★	

Date and Fig Pudding

This deliciously gingered pudding provides plenty of fibre as well as a whole selection of nutrients beneficial to the health of skin.

SERVES 4
finely grated rind and juice of 1 orange
100 g (4 oz) dried stoned dates, chopped
100 g (4 oz) dried figs, coarsely chopped

50 g (2 oz) fresh root ginger, peeled and finely shredded
25 g (1 oz) polyunsaturated margarine
25 g (1 oz) plain wholemeal flour

25 g (1 oz) plain white flour
5 ml (1 tsp) baking powder
2 eggs, beaten

150 g (5 oz) fresh wholemeal
breadcrumbs

1 Lightly grease a 900 ml (1½ pint) pudding basin.
2 Mix the orange rind and juice with the dates, figs and ginger. Set aside for 1 hour, stirring occasionally.
3 Add the margarine, flours, baking powder, eggs and breadcrumbs to the fruit mixture. Put in the basin and level the surface. Tie a pleated double thickness of greaseproof paper over the top and steam for 1½ hours or until well risen and firm to the touch. Turn out and serve with custard.

Nutritional analysis	
335 kcals/1410 kJ	7.4 mg Vitamin C ★ ★
9.9 g Protein	2.1 mcg Vitamin E ★ ★
9.4 g Fat	657 mg Potassium ★ ★
57 g Carbohydrate	126 mg Calcium ★ ★
11 g Fibre ★ ★	3.6 mg Iron ★ ★
102 mcg Vitamin A ★	

Apricot and Orange Soufflés

*A considerable amount of vitamin A is present in this dessert –
contributed by the apricots, orange, egg yolk and dairy products.
Vitamin A is believed to guard against cancers that arise in
epithelial (skin and lining) tissues.*

SERVES 4
350 g (12 oz) no-soak dried
apricots
45 ml (3 tbsp) light muscovado
sugar
3 eggs, separated
finely grated rind and juice of
1 large orange
15 ml (1 tbsp) powdered
gelatine

150 ml (¼ pint) whipping
cream
75 ml (5 tbsp) Greek-style
natural yogurt
60 ml (4 tbsp) orange-flavoured
liqueur
25 g (1 oz) flaked almonds,
toasted, to decorate

1 Prepare four 100 ml (4 fl oz) individual soufflé dishes or ramekins. Cut four strips of double greaseproof paper long enough to go around the outside of each dish, overlapping slightly and about 5 cm (2 inches) higher than the dish. Tie with string, then brush the inside of the paper above the rims with a little polyunsaturated oil. Set aside.

2 Put the apricots in a saucepan, cover with cold water and bring slowly to the boil. Lower the heat, cover and simmer for about 15 minutes or until the apricots are tender. Drain. Reserve four apricots for the decoration and purée the remainder in a blender or food processor. Set aside to cool.

3 Meanwhile, put the sugar, egg yolks and orange rind in a heatproof bowl and place over a saucepan of gently simmering water. Whisk until very thick: the beaters should leave a trail in the mixture when lifted out. Remove from the heat.

4 Sprinkle the gelatine over the orange juice in a heatproof bowl and leave to soften for 1 minute. Place over a pan of gently simmering water and stir until the gelatine has dissolved. Leave to cool slightly.

5 Lightly whip the cream and fold into the yogurt until evenly mixed. Whisk the egg whites until stiff.

6 Combine the puréed apricots and egg yolk mixture, then pour in the gelatine, stirring continuously. Mix in the liqueur. Fold in the cream and yogurt, then fold in the egg whites.

7 Divide the mixture between the prepared dishes. Chill for at least 4 hours or until set.

8 To serve, carefully remove the paper collars from the soufflés. Top each one with a reserved apricot and surround with toasted flaked almonds to form a flower shape. Finely chop the remaining almonds, then gently press around the edges of the soufflés. Serve chilled.

Nutritional analysis	
505 kcals/2105 kJ	7.2 mg Vitamin C ★ ★
15 g Protein	2.2 mcg Vitamin E ★ ★
23 g Fat	1858 mg Potassium ★ ★ ★ ★
58 g Carbohydrate	172 mg Calcium ★ ★
22 g Fibre ★ ★ ★ ★	4.9 mg Iron ★ ★ ★
724 mcg Vitamin A ★ ★ ★ ★ ★	

Apple and Lemon Sorbet

Using eating apples and no-soak dried apricots eliminates the need for added sugar in this dessert. Apart from all its other nutrients, eating apples contain surprisingly little vitamin C. Dried apricots are a good source of carotene and iron.

SERVES 4

3 red eating apples, peeled, cored and sliced
75 g (3 oz) no-soak dried apricots, rinsed and chopped

grated rind and juice of ½ lemon
300 ml (½ pint) unsweetened apple juice
2 egg whites

1 Place the apples in a blender or food processor with the apricots, lemon rind and juice and apple juice and purée until smooth.
2 Pour into a shallow freezer bowl and freeze for 45–60 minutes or until ice crystals begin to form around the edge.
3 Tip the semi-set sorbet into a bowl and beat until smooth. Whisk the egg whites until stiff but not dry, then fold into the sorbet. Return to the container and freeze for 3–4 hours or until just firm. Serve in scoops.

Nutritional analysis	
115 kcals/485 kJ	117 mcg Vitamin A ★
2.5 g Protein	4.9 mg Vitamin C ★
0 g Fat	563 mg Potassium ★
28 g Carbohydrate	1.2 mg Iron ★
6.1 g Fibre ★ ★	

Minted Strawberry Custards

Fresh strawberries contain so much vitamin C that a 100 g (4 oz) portion provides double the recommended daily amount (RDA).

SERVES 6

450 ml (¾ pint) semi-skimmed milk
4 large mint sprigs
1 whole egg
2 egg yolks
45 ml (3 tbsp) light muscovado sugar

20 ml (4 tsp) powdered gelatine
700 g (1½ lb) strawberries
polyunsaturated oil
15 ml (1 tbsp) icing sugar
a few strawberries, to decorate

1 Place the milk and mint sprigs in a saucepan. Bring slowly to the boil, then remove from the heat, cover and leave to infuse for about 30 minutes. Strain.

2 Whisk the whole egg and the yolks with the sugar and strain into the milk. Return to the pan and cook gently, stirring, until the custard just coats the back of the spoon. Do *not* boil. Leave to cool.

3 Sprinkle the gelatine over 45 ml (3 tbsp) cold water in a heatproof bowl and leave to soften for 1 minute. Place over a saucepan of gently simmering water and stir until the gelatine has dissolved. Cool slightly, then stir into the custard.

4 Purée the strawberries in a blender or food processor, then press through a sieve. Whisk about two-thirds into the cold, but not set, custard.

5 Oil six 150 ml (¼ pint) ramekin dishes. Pour in the custard and chill for about 3 hours or until set.

6 Meanwhile, whisk the icing sugar into the remaining strawberry purée and chill.

7 To serve, turn out the custards and surround with the strawberry sauce. Decorate with strawberries.

Nutritional analysis	
170 kcals/720 kJ	77 mg Vitamin C ★ ★ ★ ★ ★
8.8 g Protein	346 mg Potassium ★
6 g Fat	145 mg Calcium ★ ★
22 g Carbohydrate	1.7 mg Iron ★
0 g Fibre	

Charentais Granita

Melons and oranges, like other yellow fruit, contribute plenty of carotene for conversion into vitamin A by the body. Oranges also contribute valuable quantities of folic acid.

SERVES 4
1.6 kg (3½ lb) charentais melon, peeled, seeded and cut into chunks
15 ml (1 tbsp) clear light honey, such as Acacia

finely grated rind and juice of 1 small orange
finely grated rind and juice of 1 lemon
mint sprigs, to decorate

1 Purée the melon in a blender or food processor, then put in a bowl with the honey, rinds and juices and mix well.

2 Transfer to a freezer container and freeze for 3 hours or until the mixture is partly frozen and setting around the edges.

3 Turn the mixture into a bowl and whisk well to break up the ice crystals. Return to the container and freeze for about 4 hours or until frozen. Before serving, soften in the refrigerator for about 45 minutes. Spoon into chilled glasses or dishes and decorate with mint sprigs.

Nutritional analysis	
70 kcals/300 kJ	788 mcg Vitamin A ★ ★ ★ ★ ★
2.5 g Protein	75 mg Folic Acid ★ ★
0 g Fat	67 mg Vitamin C ★ ★ ★ ★ ★
17 g Carbohydrate	784 mg Potassium ★ ★
2.4 g Fibre	

Raspberry Bombe

This delicious and stunning-looking dessert requires only 25 ml (1½ tbsp) added sugar – use less if you wish. Main sources of vitamin B_2 (riboflavin) in the diet are milk and milk products. Deficiency can result in a host of skin disorders.

SERVES 4
225 g (8 oz) raspberries, thawed if frozen
25 ml (1½ tbsp) light muscovado sugar
10 ml (2 tsp) Crème de Cassis (blackcurrant liqueur)
225 g (8 oz) low-fat natural set yogurt
1 egg white, size 2

1 Put 175 g (6 oz) raspberries in a blender or food processor with half the sugar and the liqueur and blend to a purée. Pour into a freezerproof bowl and fold in the yogurt. Freeze for 1 hour or until ice crystals begin to form around the edge.

2 Whisk the egg white until stiff, then whisk in the remaining sugar. Remove the raspberry purée from the freezer and fold in the egg white. Pour into a 900 ml (1½ pint) decorative freezerproof mould and freeze for at least 6 hours or until frozen. Stir at least once during this time.

3 To serve, turn the bombe out of the bowl on to a serving plate and decorate with the remaining raspberries. Cut into slices.

Nutritional analysis	
80 kcals/325 kJ	4.2 g Fibre ★
4 g Protein	0.19 mg Vitamin B$_2$ ★
0.6 g Fat	14 mg Vitamin C ★ ★ ★
14 g Carbohydrate	128 mg Calcium ★ ★

Almond and Mango Ice Cream

Tofu (soya bean curd) is a very low-fat source of good quality protein. Further protein is contributed in this dish by the milk and almonds.

SERVES 8
2 medium ripe mangoes, peeled, stoned and coarsely chopped
297 g (10 oz) silken tofu
300 ml (½ pint) semi-skimmed milk
finely grated rind and juice of 1½ limes
50 g (2 oz) blanched almonds, toasted and chopped
lime slices and toasted flaked almonds, to decorate

1 Put half the mango in a blender or food processor with the tofu, milk and lime rind and juice. Blend well until smooth.
2 Pour the mixture into a shallow freezer container and freeze for about 2 hours or until ice crystals form around the edges.
3 Turn into a large, chilled bowl and mash the ice crystals with a fork. Fold in the remaining mango and the chopped almonds. Return to the freezer and freeze for 3–4 hours or until firm.
4 About 30 minutes before serving, remove from the freezer and leave the ice cream to soften at room temperature. Serve decorated with lime slices and toasted flaked almonds.

Nutritional analysis	
170 kcals/710 kJ	120 mg Calcium ★ ★
4.2 g Protein	190 mcg Vitamin A ★ ★
12 g Fat	19.5 mg Vitamin C ★ ★ ★ ★
12.5 g Carbohydrate	1.8 mcg Vitamin E ★
2 g Fibre	

Walnut Pear Slice

*Walnuts and polyunsaturated margarine are sources of vitamin E.
Grind walnuts through a nut mouli or in a food processor until fine
but not oily.*

SERVES 4
50 g (2 oz) plain white flour
50 g (2 oz) plain wholemeal flour
2.5 ml (½ tsp) ground cinnamon
25 g (1 oz) ground walnuts
finely grated rind and juice of
½ lemon
1 egg

50 g (2 oz) light muscovado
sugar
50 g (2 oz) polyunsaturated
margarine
45 ml (3 tbsp) fresh wholemeal
breadcrumbs
3 ripe pears

1 Sift the flours with the cinnamon on to a clean dry work surface,
adding any bran remaining in the sieve. Sprinkle the walnuts and
lemon rind over the flour.
2 Make a well in the centre and break in the egg. Add the sugar
and margarine. With the fingertips of one hand only, pinch the
ingredients from the well together until evenly blended. Draw in
the flour gradually, with the help of a palette knife, and knead to a
smooth dough. Wrap and chill for about 30 minutes.
3 Roll out the pastry on a lightly floured surface to an oblong about
30.5 × 10 cm (12 × inches). Lift the pastry on to a baking sheet and
sprinkle over the breadcrumbs.
4 Peel, quarter and core the pears. Slice each quarter into four or
five pieces and toss gently in the lemon juice. Drain and arrange in
overlapping lines across the dough.
5 Bake at 190°C (375°F) mark 5 for about 30 minutes or until the
pastry is well browned and crisp around the edges. Allow to cool
slightly. Cut into slices and serve with yogurt.

Nutritional analysis	
315 kcals/1315 kJ	114 mcg Vitamin A ★
4.8 g Protein	3.6 mg Vitamin C ★
14 g Fat	3.3 mcg Vitamin E ★ ★
45 g Carbohydrate	1.6 mg Iron ★
4.9 g Fibre ★	

Rhubarb Brown Betty

Whole-grain products, such as wholemeal bread, contain more potassium than their refined counterparts. The rhubarb and orange juice in this dessert contribute further amounts.

SERVES 4
450 g (1 lb) rhubarb
225 g (8 oz) fresh wholemeal breadcrumbs
50 g (2 oz) light muscovado sugar

2.5 ml (½ tsp) ground ginger
50 ml (2 fl oz) unsweetened orange juice

1 Trim the rhubarb and cut the stalks into short lengths. Put in a greased 900 ml (1½ pint) ovenproof dish.
2 Mix the breadcrumbs, sugar and ground ginger together and sprinkle over the fruit. Spoon the orange juice over the crumbs.
3 Bake in the oven at 170°C (325°F) mark 3 for 40 minutes or until the fruit is soft and the topping browned. Serve hot or cold, with natural yogurt.

Nutritional analysis	
185 kcals/770 kJ	18 mg Vitamin C ★ ★ ★
5.8 g Protein	647 mg Potassium ★ ★
1.5 g Fat	134 mg Calcium ★ ★
39 g Carbohydrate	2.1 mg Iron ★
7.7 g Fibre ★ ★	

Gooseberry and Plum Tart

The wholemeal flour and fresh fruit in this tart contribute different forms of dietary fibre – insoluble cereal fibre and soluble pectin found in fruit.

MAKES 8 SLICES
100 g (4 oz) plain wholemeal flour
2.5 ml (½ tsp) cream of tartar
1.25 ml (¼ tsp) bicarbonate of soda
50 g (2 oz) polyunsaturated margarine
45 ml (3 tbsp) light muscovado sugar

1 egg yolk
15 ml (1 tbsp) semi-skimmed milk
700 g (1½ lb) ripe plums, halved, stoned and quartered
175 g (6 oz) ripe gooseberries, topped and tailed
30 ml (2 tbsp) ginger wine
5 ml (1 tsp) powdered gelatine

1 Lightly grease a 23 cm (9 inch) fluted loose-based flan tin or ring and set aside. Sift the flour, cream of tartar and bicarbonate of soda into a bowl.

2 Add the margarine and rub in lightly, then stir in 15 ml (1 tbsp) sugar. Add the egg yolk and milk and mix to a smooth dough. Press the dough into the prepared tin, shaping it up the sides to form a rim. Chill for 30 minutes.

3 Arrange the plum quarters, skin side up, in the flan case. Sprinkle with 15 ml (1 tbsp) sugar. Bake at 190°C (375°F) mark 5 for 30 minutes. Leave to cool.

4 Meanwhile, put the gooseberries, wine and remaining sugar in a saucepan with 45 ml (3 tbsp) water. Simmer for 5 minutes, then cool and sieve.

5 Sprinkle the gelatine over 30 ml (2 tbsp) cold water and leave to soften for 1 minute. Place over a saucepan of gently simmering water and stir until the gelatine has dissolved. Cool slightly, then stir into the gooseberry mixture. Spoon the gooseberry glaze evenly over the plums and leave to chill for about 2 hours before serving.

Nutritional analysis Per Slice	
165 kcals/685 kJ	107 mcg Vitamin A ★
3.5 g Protein	0.12 mg Vitamin B$_1$ ★
6.4 g Fat	11 mg Vitamin C ★ ★
23 g Carbohydrate	2.6 mcg Vitamin E ★ ★
3.7 g Fibre ★	

Baked Apple and Coconut Pudding

Pectin, a soluble form of dietary fibre found in apples, and polyunsaturated fatty acids in margarine, both help to lower blood cholesterol levels. High blood cholesterol raises the risk of developing coronary heart disease.

SERVES 6
100 g (4 oz) light muscovado sugar
100 g (4 oz) polyunsaturated margarine
finely grated rind of 1 lemon
2 eggs, separated
100 g (4 oz) plain wholemeal flour

7.5 ml (1½ tsp) baking powder
25 g (1 oz) desiccated coconut
6 medium eating apples, each weighing about 100 g (4 oz)
60 ml (4 tbsp) lemon juice
60 ml (4 tbsp) reduced-sugar apricot jam
toasted shredded coconut, to decorate

1 Beat together the sugar and margarine until well blended. Add the lemon rind, then beat in the egg yolks one at a time. Fold in the flour, baking powder and desiccated coconut.

2 Peel and core the apples, keeping them whole, and brush with 45 ml (3 tbsp) lemon juice.

3 Whisk the egg whites until stiff but not dry and fold into the creamed ingredients. Spoon into a lightly greased 24–25.5 cm (9½–10 inch) fluted flan dish. Press the apples into the mixture, spooning a little of the remaining lemon juice over them.

4 Stand the dish on a baking sheet and bake at 170°C (325°F) mark 3 for 1–1¼ hours or until well browned and firm to the touch, covering lightly if necessary. Leave to cool for about 15 minutes.

5 Put the jam and remaining lemon juice in a small saucepan and heat gently, stirring, until the jam softens. Bring to the boil and simmer for 1 minute. Brush the dessert with the apricot glaze and scatter over the shredded coconut. Serve warm.

Nutritional analysis	
430 kcals/1795 kJ	218 mcg Vitamin A ★
5.1 g Protein	5.5 mg Vitamin C ★
22 g Fat	5.8 mcg Vitamin E ★ ★
56 g Carbohydrate	1.7 mg Iron ★
3.9 g Fibre ★	

12
Baking

Foods rich in important nutrients, such as fruit, nuts and seeds, can be included in a wide variety of breads, cakes, teabreads and biscuits. Cakes need not be sickly sweet and filled with whipped cream to be delicious. The Spicy Apple Cake overleaf contains little sugar and is flavoured with mixed spice and apples for sweetness. The Pear and Nut Cake is sweetened with honey. The breads at the end of the chapter are packed with goodness; don't spoil it by covering slices with a thick layer of butter – use polyunsaturated margarine instead.

Spicy Apple Cake

Incorporating dried dates into this cake allows for a reduction in the amount of added sugar needed, whilst increasing the fibre content, making it a much healthier teatime favourite.

MAKES 6 SLICES
225 g (8 oz) plain wholemeal flour
10 ml (2 tsp) baking powder
5 ml (1 tsp) ground mixed spice
100 g (4 oz) light muscovado sugar

100 g (4 oz) polyunsaturated margarine
75 g (3 oz) stoned dried dates, chopped
2 eggs, size 2, beaten
450 g (1 lb) cooking apples, peeled, cored and diced

1 Put the flour, baking powder, mixed spice and sugar in a bowl. Rub in the margarine, then add the dates and beaten eggs.
2 Carefully fold three-quarters of the apple into the mixture. Spoon into a greased and floured deep round 20.5 cm (8 inch) loose-bottomed cake tin and smooth the top.
3 Scatter the remaining apple over the cake. Bake at 180°C (350°F) mark 4 for 1¼–1½ hours or until risen, golden brown and cooked through. Cover with greaseproof paper after 50 minutes to prevent overbrowning.
4 Cool in the tin before turning out and serving cut into slices.

Nutritional analysis Per Slice	
365 kcals/1530 kJ	180 mcg Vitamin A ★
7.7 g Protein	12 mg Vitamin C ★ ★
16 g Fat	5 mcg Vitamin E ★ ★ ★
51 g Carbohydrate	2.4 mg Iron ★ ★
5.6 g Fibre ★	

Pear and Nut Cake

The use of polyunsaturated margarine instead of butter reduces the amount of saturated fat in this cake. Diets high in saturated fat are linked to an increased risk of coronary heart disease.

MAKES 8 SLICES
4 dessert pears (about 550 g/1¼ lb total weight), peeled and cored

75 g (3 oz) polyunsaturated margarine
45 ml (3 tbsp) clear honey
2 eggs, beaten

100 g (4 oz) self-raising
wholemeal flour
100 g (4 oz) self-raising white
flour

5 ml (1 tsp) baking powder
5 ml (1 tsp) ground mace
50 g (2 oz) shelled walnuts,
chopped

1 Grease and line an 18 cm (7 inch) round cake tin. Purée three of the pears in a blender or food processor until smooth. Thinly slice the remaining pear and reserve.

2 Cream the margarine and honey together, then gradually add the eggs with a little flour, beating well after each addition. Sift the baking powder and mace together. Fold into the mixture together with the remaining flour and the walnuts. Mix in the pear purée.

3 Put half the mixture in the prepared tin, lay the reserved pear slices on top and cover with the remaining mixture. Bake at 190°C (375°F) mark 5 for about 1 hour or until a skewer inserted in the centre of the cake comes out clean. Cool in the tin before turning out. Leave until the next day before slicing.

Nutritional analysis Per Slice	
240 kcals/1005 kJ	105 mcg Vitamin A ★
5.4 g Protein	2.7 mcg Vitamin E ★ ★
13 g Fat	64 mg Calcium ★
28 g Carbohydrate	1.4 mg Iron ★
3.2 g Fibre ★	

Spiced Fruit Cake

An oil-based fruit cake with a delicious crumbly texture. For a firmer texture use half wholemeal and half white flour. Iron and vitamin E are the two most plentiful nutrients in this cake.

MAKES 14 SLICES
250 g (9 oz) prunes, rinsed
175 g (6 oz) glacé cherries,
roughly chopped
250 g (9 oz) sultanas, rinsed
40 g (1½ oz) mixed peel
30 ml (2 tbsp) whisky
450 g (1 lb) plain wholemeal
flour
20 ml (4 tsp) baking powder

10 ml (2 tsp) ground mixed
spice
175 g (6 oz) dark muscovado
sugar
300 ml (½ pint)
polyunsaturated oil
4 eggs, lightly beaten
60 ml (4 tbsp) semi-skimmed
milk

1 Snip the prunes into small pieces, discarding the stones. Put the prunes and cherries in a bowl with the sultanas and mixed peel. Stir in the whisky, cover and leave to stand in a cool place overnight.

2 Grease and line the base and sides of a 20.5 cm (8 inch) square cake tin.

3 Place the flour, baking powder, spice and sugar in a bowl. Make a well in the centre and add the oil, eggs and milk. Beat well for about 3 minutes until very smooth. Stir in the fruit and spoon into the prepared tin.

4 Bake at 170°C (325°F) mark 3 for 1 hour, then reduce the heat to 150°C (300°F) mark 2 and bake for a further 1¼ hours, or until the cake is cooked and a skewer inserted in the centre of the cake comes out clean. Cover the cake with kitchen foil to prevent overbrowning towards the end of cooking, if necessary.

5 Allow the cake to cool in the tin. Turn out, then wrap in greaseproof paper and foil and leave for 2–3 days to mature.

Nutritional analysis Per Slice	
480 kcals/2015 kJ	0.2 mg Vitamin B₁ ★
7.3 g Protein	11 mcg Vitamin E ★ ★ ★ ★ ★
24 g Fat	3 mg Iron ★ ★
61 g Carbohydrate	1.2 mg Zinc ★
7.3 g Fibre ★ ★	

Cottage Cheese and Brazil Nut Teabread

This recipe uses cottage cheese instead of margarine or butter which reduces the overall fat content. Serve cold, spread thinly with a little polyunsaturated margarine, if liked.

MAKES 15 SLICES
225 g (8 oz) cottage cheese
75 g (3 oz) light muscovado sugar
225 g (8 oz) self-raising wholemeal flour
finely grated rind and juice of 1 lemon
2 eggs, beaten
75 ml (5 tbsp) semi-skimmed milk
75 g (3 oz) stoned dried dates, rinsed and roughly chopped
75 g (3 oz) Brazil nuts, chopped
6 whole Brazil nuts, to decorate
15 ml (1 tbsp) clear honey, to glaze

1 Grease and base-line a 900 g (2 lb) loaf tin and set aside. Put all the ingredients, except the whole Brazil nuts and honey, in a bowl and beat well together until the mixture has a soft dropping consistency.

2 Spoon into the prepared tin and level the surface. Lightly press the whole Brazil nuts in a line down the centre of the mixture to decorate.

3 Bake at 180°C (350°F) mark 4 for 50–60 minutes or until risen and golden brown, covering with greaseproof paper if the teabread is browning too quickly. Turn out and brush with the honey while still warm. Leave to cool on a wire rack.

Nutritional analysis Per Slice	
160 kcals/665 kJ	0.16 mg Vitamin B₁ ★
6.2 g Protein	183 mg Potassium
6.6 g Fat	45 mg Calcium
20 g Carbohydrate	1.1 mg Iron
2.6 g Fibre	

Apricot Oat Crunchies

These delicious chewy teatime bars will become a firm favourite. They are also very good for you, containing fibre and vitamins A and E.

MAKES 12
75 g (3 oz) self-raising wholemeal flour
75 g (3 oz) rolled (porridge) oats
75 g (3 oz) light muscovado sugar
100 g (4 oz) polyunsaturated margarine
100 g (4 oz) no-soak dried apricots, chopped

1 Lightly grease a shallow oblong baking tin measuring 28 × 18 × 3.5 cm (11 × 7 × 1½ inches).

2 Mix together the flour, oats and sugar in a bowl and rub in the margarine until the mixture resembles breadcrumbs.

3 Spread half the oat mixture over the base of the prepared tin, pressing it down evenly. Spread the apricots over the oat mixture, then sprinkle over the remaining mixture and press down well.

4 Bake in the oven at 180°C (350°F) mark 4 for 25 minutes or until golden brown. Leave in the tin for about 1 hour or until cold. Cut into bars to serve.

Nutritional analysis Per Bar	
145 kcals/610 kJ	125 mcg Vitamin A ★
2 g Protein	2.2 mcg Vitamin E ★ ★
7.4 g Fat	208 mg Potassium
19 g Carbohydrate	0.9 mg Iron
3 g Fibre ★	

Strawberry and Passion Fruit Swiss Roll

Swiss rolls are low in fat, and this one runs true to form with a delicious low-fat filling.

SERVES 6
3 eggs
100 g (4 oz) light muscovado sugar
50 g (2 oz) plain wholemeal flour
50 g (2 oz) plain white flour

finely grated rind of 1 lemon
caster sugar
225 g (8 oz) strawberries, hulled
2 passion fruit
150 g (5 oz) low-fat soft cheese

1 Grease and base-line a 33 × 23 × 2 cm (13 × 9 × ¾ inch) Swiss roll tin.
2 Using an electric mixer, whisk the eggs and sugar together until very thick and pale. (The mixture should leave a trail when the beaters are lifted from the bowl.) Carefully fold in the flours and lemon rind, then gently stir in 15 ml (1 tbsp) water. Pour the mixture into the prepared tin.
3 Bake at 200°C (400°F) mark 6 for about 12 minutes or until golden brown and just firm to the touch.
4 As soon as the cake is out of the oven, run a blunt-edged knife around the edges of the sponge and sprinkle the top with caster sugar. Cover with a sheet of greaseproof paper and a baking sheet. Invert and carefully lift the tin off the sponge.
5 Trim the crusty edges of the sponge, then make a shallow cut across one of the narrow ends. Roll up from this end, rolling the paper inside the sponge. Leave to cool.

6 Meanwhile, mash half the strawberries and roughly chop the remainder. Halve the passion fruit and scoop out the flesh. Beat together the low-fat cheese with the scooped-out passion fruit flesh. Stir in the mashed strawberries.

7 Carefully unroll the sponge, removing the paper. Spread the filling over the surface and spoon over the strawberry pieces. Roll up again, cover and chill lightly before serving. This roll is best eaten on the same day it is made.

Nutritional analysis	
225 kcals/940 kJ	0.21 mg Vitamin B₁ ★
9 g Protein	24 mg Vitamin C ★ ★ ★ ★
5.5 g Fat	66 mg Calcium ★
37 g Carbohydrate	1.7 mg Iron ★
3.5 g Fibre ★	

Fruit Teabread

This is a very low-fat teabread, with plenty of energy provided by the carbohydrate. A subtle change of flavour could be made by varying the type of tea used; try Earl Grey, Darjeeling or rosehip.

MAKES 8 SLICES
300 ml (½ pint) cold tea
100 g (4 oz) seedless raisins
100 g (4 oz) sultanas
100 g (4 oz) chopped mixed peel, well rinsed
1 egg, beaten

75 g (3 oz) plain wholemeal flour
75 g (3 oz) plain white flour
50 g (2 oz) light muscovado sugar
5 ml (1 tsp) baking powder

1 Mix together the tea, raisins, sultanas and mixed peel and leave to soak for at least 8 hours or overnight.

2 Lightly grease and line a 450 g (1 lb) loaf tin. Add the egg, flours, sugar and baking powder to the tea and fruit. Mix well and pour into the tin.

3 Bake at 180°C (350°F) mark 4 for 1 hour or until the loaf pulls away from the sides of the tin and feels firm to the touch. Turn out on to a wire rack and leave to cool completely. Serve sliced.

Nutritional analysis Per Slice	
185 kcals/780 kJ	3 g Fibre ★
3.5 g Protein	286 mg Potassium
1.1 g Fat	44 mg Calcium
44 g Carbohydrate	1.6 mg Iron ★

Sunflower Flapjacks

The fibre found in oats helps to prevent the excessive rise of blood cholesterol, high levels of which are associated with heart disease. Vitamin E, also present in these flapjacks, helps to prevent fluid retention and is also associated with the fight against heart disease. Use the jumbo oats available from healthfood shops; porridge oats give a softer texture.

MAKES 12
275 g (10 oz) rolled oats
100 g (4 oz) sunflower seeds
100 g (4 oz) polyunsaturated margarine
75 ml (5 tbsp) golden syrup

1 Place the oats and sunflower seeds in a bowl and make a well in the centre. Heat the margarine and syrup in a saucepan until melted and evenly blended, then pour into the well.
2 Stir the mixture until the oats and seeds are evenly coated, then spoon into a 27 × 17.5 × 3.5 cm (10¾ × 7 × 1⅜ inch) shallow cake tin. Press down well with the back of a spoon.
3 Bake at 180°C (350°F) mark 4 for about 35 minutes or until golden brown and just firm to the touch.
4 Allow to cool completely in the tin, then cut into small triangles.

Nutritional analysis Per Flapjack	
240 kcals/1000 kJ	94 mcg Vitamin A ★
4.6 g Protein	2.8 mcg Vitamin E ★ ★
14 g Fat	1.7 mg Iron ★
26 g Carbohydrate	185 mg Potassium
2 g Fibre	

Crumbly Muesli Bars

Consuming 35–45 g (1¼–1½ oz) oats or oatmeal per day, on top of a reduced-fat diet, has a definite lowering effect on blood cholesterol – thus reducing the risk of a heart attack.

MAKES 14

275 g (10 oz) unsweetened muesli

50 g (2 oz) plain wholemeal flour

2.5 ml (½ tsp) baking powder

2.5 ml (½ tsp) ground cinnamon

100 g (4 oz) polyunsaturated margarine

25 g (1 oz) light muscovado sugar

45 ml (3 tbsp) semi-skimmed milk

45 ml (3 tbsp) reduced-sugar blackcurrant jam

1 Place the muesli, flour, baking powder and cinnamon in a bowl. Add the margarine and work into the dry ingredients with a fork.

2 Stir in the sugar, then add the milk. Stir until the mixture begins to come together.

3 Press half the mixture into a lightly greased 27 × 17.5 × 3.5 cm (10¾ × 7 × 1⅜ inch) shallow cake tin. Spread the jam over, then top with the remaining muesli mixture, pressing down well. Chill for about 15 minutes.

4 Bake at 190°C (375°F) mark 5 for about 30 minutes or until firm to the touch and golden brown.

5 Leave to cool slightly in the tin, then cut into thin fingers and remove from the tin. Place on a wire rack to cool completely.

Nutritional analysis Per Bar	
160 kcals/670 kJ	81 mcg Vitamin A ★
2.5 g Protein	2.9 mcg Vitamin E ★ ★
8.5 g Fat	53 mg Calcium ★
20 g Carbohydrate	1.2 mg Iron ★
1.8 g Fibre	

Sesame Seed Biscuits

Although the amount of nutrients in each biscuit does not rate a star, they are valuable nutrients which all contribute to one's over-all intake.

MAKES 20
100 g (4 oz) polyunsaturated margarine
50 g (2 oz) light muscovado sugar
grated rind of 1 orange
50 g (2 oz) walnuts, finely chopped

50 g (2 oz) no-soak dried apricots, rinsed and finely chopped
75 g (3 oz) sesame seeds
1 egg, beaten
40 g (1½ oz) plain wholemeal flour
40 g (1½ oz) plain white flour

1 Lightly grease a baking sheet. Heat the margarine and sugar together in a saucepan until the sugar has dissolved. Stir in the orange rind, walnuts, apricots and sesame seeds. Add the egg and flours and mix well.

2 Drop small dessertspoons of the mixture on to the baking sheet, leaving enough space between to allow for spreading. Bake at 190°C (375°F) mark 5 for 15 minutes or until pale golden. Leave to cool for a few minutes on the baking sheet, then transfer to a wire rack to cool completely.

Nutritional analysis Per Biscuit	
105 kcals/435 kJ	1.3 mcg Vitamin E
1.9 g Protein	98 mg Potassium
7.8 g Fat	47 mg Calcium
7.5 g Carbohydrate	0.9 mg Iron
1.2 g Fibre	

Peanut Cookies

What appears to be small amounts of nutrients in these biscuits all add up, e.g. two cookies will contribute 1 mg of iron which is a notable amount. Choose a peanut butter with no added sugar, available mainly from healthfood shops.

MAKES 20
50 g (2 oz) polyunsaturated margarine

75 g (3 oz) crunchy peanut butter
50 g (2 oz) light muscovado sugar

1 egg
150 g (5 oz) plain wholemeal
flour

2.5 ml (½ tsp) baking powder
50 g (2 oz) shelled unsalted
peanuts, roughly chopped

1 Beat together the margarine, peanut butter, sugar and egg until evenly blended. Stir in the flour and baking powder.
2 Roll the mixture into small balls (about the size of walnuts) in your hands until smooth. Place well apart on baking sheets and flatten lightly with a fork. Chill for about 15 minutes.
3 Sprinkle some chopped peanuts over each biscuit. Bake at 190°C (375°F) mark 5 for about 12 minutes or until pale golden.
4 Allow to cool for about 5 minutes to firm up slightly, then transfer to a wire rack to cool completely.

Nutritional analysis Per Cookie	
95 kcals/395 kJ	1.1 mcg Vitamin E
2.8 g Protein	77 mg Potassium
5.7 g Fat	0.5 mg Iron
8.3 g Carbohydrate	0.45 mg Zinc
1.2 g Fibre	

Granary and Walnut French Sticks

Both vitamin B_1 and folic acid (which is also a B vitamin) are fragile water-soluble vitamins often lost during food preparation. Vitamin B_1 is essential for energy production from carbohydrate as well as for maintaining a healthy skin.

MAKES 12 SLICES
450 g (1 lb) strong granary flour
1 sachet easy mix dried yeast
50 g (2 oz) walnut halves,
chopped

5 ml (1 tsp) salt
1 egg, beaten

1 Mix together the flour, yeast, walnuts and salt. Make a well in the centre and add 300 ml (½ pint) tepid water. Mix to a soft dough. Turn out on to a lightly floured surface and knead the dough for about 10 minutes or until smooth and no longer sticky.

2 Divide the dough in two and roll out each piece to a 30.5 × 15 cm (12 × 6 inch) rectangle. Roll up each from the longest edge and place seam-side down on floured baking sheets.
3 Make shallow slashes along each loaf. Cover with a clean cloth and leave in a warm place for about 1 hour or until doubled in size. Brush lightly with beaten egg.
4 Place a roasting tin half filled with water in the bottom of the oven, then bake the bread at 220°C (425°F) mark 7 for about 15 minutes. Remove the roasting tin and bake the French sticks for a further 8 minutes or until well browned and hollow- sounding when tapped.

Nutritional analysis Per Slice	
155 kcals/655 kJ	61.8 mg Calcium ★
6 g Protein	1.6 mg Iron ★
3.8 g Fat	0.18 mg Vitamin B$_1$ ★
26 g Carbohydrate	48 mg Folic Acid ★
3.1 g Fibre ★	

Mixed Grain Bread

Whole grains are an excellent source of high-fibre unrefined carbo-hydrate. The body converts all carbohydrate into 'simple' sugars which are then used as an energy source.

MAKES 2 LOAVES, ABOUT
30 SLICES
100 g (4 oz) whole wheat grain
100 g (4 oz) millet
900 g (2 lb) granary flour
50 g (2 oz) rolled oats
25 g (1 oz) wheatgerm

30 ml (2 tbsp) sunflower seeds
7.5 ml (1½ tsp) salt
1 sachet easy mix dried yeast
finely grated rind and juice of
2 oranges
30 ml (2 tbsp) polyunsaturated
oil

1 Lightly grease two baking sheets. Put the whole wheat grain and millet in a bowl. Pour over boiling water to cover and leave to soak until the grains soften.
2 Meanwhile, put the flour, oats, wheatgerm, sunflower seeds, salt and yeast in a large bowl and mix together. Stir in the orange rind and juice and oil. Add about 600 ml (1 pint) warm water and

mix to form a firm, pliable dough that leaves the sides of the bowl clean.

3 Turn the dough out on to a lightly floured surface and knead for about 10 minutes or until smooth and elastic.

4 Shape into a ball, return to the bowl and cover with a clean cloth. Leave to rise in a warm place for about 1 hour or until doubled in size.

5 Drain the soaked grains very well. Turn the dough on to a lightly floured surface and knead the grains into the dough. Knead for a further 2–3 minutes, then divide the dough in half and shape each portion into a ball.

6 Flatten each ball, then roll up like a Swiss roll. Tuck the edges under and place on the baking sheets.

7 Cover with a clean cloth and leave to prove in a warm place for about 30 minutes or until doubled in size.

8 Bake at 200°C (400°F) mark 6 for 30–40 minutes or until risen and golden brown, and the loaves sound hollow when tapped on the base. Switch the position of the baking sheets on the oven shelves halfway through the cooking time. Cool on a wire rack.

Nutritional analysis Per Slice	
145 kcals/605 kJ	0.19 mg Vitamin B_1 ★
5.3 g Protein	34 mg Folic Acid ★
2.3 g Fat	50 mg Calcium ★
27 g Carbohydrate	1.7 mg Iron ★
3 g Fibre ★	

Flowerpot Loaves

The unusual shape of these loaves intrigues children – this will encourage them to eat this high-fibre bread which can be made into round sandwiches.

MAKES 3 LOAVES
1 sachet easy mix dried yeast
700 g (1½ lb) plain wholemeal flour

25 g (1 oz) soya flour
7.5 ml (1½ tsp) salt
milk or water, to glaze
cracked wheat

1 Choose three clean, new 10–12.5 cm (4–5 inch) clay flowerpots. Before using for the first time, grease well and bake in a hot oven for about 30 minutes. This stops the flowerpots cracking and the loaves sticking. Leave to cool, then grease again.

2 Mix the yeast, flours and salt in a bowl and make a well in the centre. Pour in 600 ml (1 pint) tepid water and mix to a soft dough that leaves the bowl clean. Turn the dough on to a lightly floured surface and knead thoroughly for about 10 minutes or until smooth and elastic.

3 Divide the dough into three and shape to fit the greased flowerpots. Cover with a clean cloth and leave in a warm place for about 1 hour or until doubled in size.

4 Brush the tops lightly with milk or water and sprinkle with cracked wheat. Bake in the oven at 230°C (450°F) mark 8 for 15 minutes, then reduce the oven temperature to 200°C (400°F) mark 6 and bake for a further 30–40 minutes or until the loaves are well risen and firm. Turn out and leave to cool on a wire rack for about 1 hour before slicing and spreading.

Nutritional analysis Per Loaf	
780 kcals/3255 kJ	104 mg Calcium
35 g Protein	11 mg Iron
5.3 g Fat	7.2 mg Zinc
157 g Carbohydrate	1.2 mg Thiamin
24 g Fibre	233 mg Folic Acid
1059 mg Potassium	

Club Sandwiches

These sandwiches provide a good quantity of zinc – one of the minerals that is often deficient in diets. A good zinc intake is important for many things in the body, including healthy hair.

SERVES 2
30 ml (2 tbsp) thick low-fat natural yogurt
15 ml (1 tbsp) mayonnaise
1 gherkin, finely chopped
1 small garlic clove, skinned and crushed

2.5 ml (½ tsp) mild mustard
salt and pepper
6 slices of wholemeal bread
a few lettuce leaves
2 thick slices of cooked turkey
2 large tomatoes, sliced
2 slices of lean ham

1 Mix together the yogurt, mayonnaise, gherkin, garlic, mustard and salt and pepper to taste.

2 Toast the bread on both sides and spread one side of each slice with the yogurt dressing. Arrange half the lettuce leaves on two slices of toast and top with the turkey. Season to taste with pepper, then add another slice of toast to each, dressing-side upwards.

3 Arrange the remaining lettuce on top with the tomato and ham. Top with the remaining toast slice, dressing-side down.

4 Cut each sandwich diagonally into quarters and secure each quarter with a cocktail stick. Arrange, crust-side down on two plates.

Nutritional analysis	
440 kcals/1835 kJ	149 mcg Vitamin A ★ ★
30 g Protein	27 mg Vitamin C ★ ★ ★ ★ ★
12 g Fat	920 mg Potassium ★ ★
56 g Carbohydrate	4.6 mg Iron ★ ★
12 g Fibre ★ ★	4.5 mg Zinc ★ ★

Index

abscesses, 61
acne, 8–9, 12, 22, 27, 28, 29, 59
acne rosacea, 18, 27, 55, 59–60
additives, 55–6
adrenal glands, 21, 30
ageing, 16, 17, 24–5, 54, 60
AIDS, 12
alcohol, 8, 15, 23, 24–6, 45
allergies, 12, 13–14, 15, 18, 29, 53,
    54–6
almonds: almond and mango
    ice cream, 218
    mackerel fillets in oatmeal and
    almonds, 131
alpha-linolenic acid, 50–51
amino acids, 46–7
androgens, 8–9
antibiotics, 27–8
antigen presenting (AP) cells, 3
apples: apple and lemon sorbet, 215
    baked apple and coconut pudding,
    221–2
    curried apple coleslaw, 190–91
    spicy apple cake, 224
apricots: apricot and orange soufflés,
    213–14
    apricot and redcurrant stuffed
    pork, 147–8
    apricot oat crunchies, 227–8
arachidonic acid, 49, 51
ascorbic acid see vitamin C
Asian skin, 5–6, 20
asparagus: asparagus with
    orange sauce, 100–101
    stir-fried asparagus, 181
atopic eczema, 12, 50
aubergines: aubergine and bean
    gratin, 119–20
    chicken Parmigiana, 152
    ratatouille cheese pie, 167–8
    stuffed baked aubergines, 168–9

avocado: avocado and chick-peas
    salad, 122
    avocado soup, 94
    bean, cheese and avocado salad,
    196
    chicken and avocado Stroganoff,
    155
    crab-stuffed avocado, 103–4

bacon: brown rice with kidney and
    bacon, 82–3
bananas: barbecued bananas, 207
    cauliflower, banana and date salad,
    194
barbecue dishes, 199–208
barbecued bananas, 207
barbecued red mullet, 205
basil and tomato tartlets, 101–2
bass baked in mint, 129
bean and chicken tabouleh, 112
bean, cheese and avocado salad, 196
bean sprouts: haddock and prawn
    stir-fry, 134
    Oriental salad, 191–2
    sprouted salad, 195
beef: beef braised in beer, 145
    beef Burgundy, 144
    hamburgers, 202
beer, beef braised in, 145
biotin, 36
biscuits: peanut cookies, 232–3
    sesame seed biscuits, 232
black beans and rice, 158
black skins, 6, 20
blackcurrant sauce, pears with, 211
blood system, 4, 11
blue cheese dip, 123
boils, 61
bombe, raspberry, 217–18
Brazil nuts: cottage cheese and Brazil
    nut teabread, 226–7

bread: club sandwiches, 236–7
  flowerpot loaves, 235–6
  granary and walnut French sticks,
    233–4
  mixed grain bread, 234–5
  nut soda bread, 80–81
breakfast, 75–87
broken red veins, 5, 26, 61–2
brown rice with kidney and bacon,
  82–3
bruises, 62
brunch, 75–87
Brussels sprouts with hazelnuts, 178
bulgar wheat: bean and chicken
    tabouleh, 112
  bulgar kedgeree, 86–7
  mixed grain and nut salad, 197–8
burdock, great, 56–7
burns, 62

caffeine, 17, 26–7
cakes: pear and nut cake, 224–5
  spiced fruit cake, 225–6
  spicy apple cake, 224
  strawberry and passion fruit Swiss
    roll, 228–9
calcium, 38, 40
cancer, 18–19
candidiasis, 53, 70–71
cannellini beans: aubergine and bean
    gratin, 119–20
carotene see vitamin A
carrots: roasted oatmeal vegetables,
  176–7
  vegetable curry, 162
cashew nuts: mushroom and cashew
    toasts, 85–6
cauliflower: cauliflower and courgette
    bake, 169–70
  cauliflower, banana and date salad,
    194
celeriac: celeriac salad, 186–7
  celeriac with tomato sauce, 174
chamomile, German, 57
chapped skin, 63
charentais granita, 216–17
cheese: baked jacket potatoes with
    hummus, 121
  basil and tomato tartlets, 101–2
  bean, cheese and avocado salad,
    196

cheese (cont'd)
  chicken Parmigiana, 152
  cottage cheese and Brazil nut
    teabread, 224–7
  goat's cheese tarts, 120
  grape, watercress and Stilton salad,
    188
  nut and cheese plait, 166–7
  pasta shells with cheese and
    walnuts, 164
  ratatouille cheese pie, 167–8
  spinach and cheese quiche with
    crisp potato crust, 118–19
  yogurt dips with crudités, 123
cherries: red cherry soup, 95
chick-peas: avocado and chick-peas
    salad, 122
  baked jacket potatoes with hummus,
    121
chicken: bean and chicken tabouleh,
    112
  chicken and avocado Stroganoff,
    155
  chicken and grape salad, 187–8
  chicken and orange kebabs, 154
  chicken Parmigiana, 152
  honeyed chicken, 151
  mustard chicken drumsticks, 204–5
  raspberry chicken with peaches,
    150–51
  smoked chicken and mint salad,
    105–6
  tandoori chicken, 206
chives, sautéed courgettes with, 175
chloasma, 9, 28, 35
choline, 36
chowder, sweetcorn and haddock, 97
circulatory system, 10–11
cis-linoleic acid, 26, 49
club sandwiches, 236–7
cockles: mixed seafood salad, 137–8
  seafood spaghetti, 113
coconut: baked apple and coconut
    pudding, 221–2
  curried fish with coconut, 133–4
coffee, 23, 26–7, 43
cold sores, 63
cold weather, 15
coleslaw, curried apple, 190–91
coley: curried fish with coconut,
    133–4

collagen, 4, 10, 17, 25
comfrey, 57
Continental dip, 123
contraceptive pill, 28–9
cooking methods, 52
copper, 43
coriander noodles, 143
corticosteriods, 29–30
cottage cheese and Brazil nut
        teabread, 226–7
courgettes: cauliflower and courgette
        bake, 169–170
    coriander noodles, 163
    courgette and pepper salad, 190
    ratatouille cheese pie, 167–8
    sautéed courgettes with chives, 175
    vegetable curry, 162
crab: crab-stuffed avocado, 103
    mixed seafood salad, 137–8
cross-linking, 15–16, 24, 54
crumbly muesli bars, 231
crunchy winter salad, 184–5
cucumber: cold cucumber soup, 93–4
    stir-fried kippers and cucumber,
        115–16
curries: curried apple coleslaw,
        190–91
    curried fish with coconut, 133–4
    vegetable curry, 162
custards, minted strawberry, 215–16
cuts, 71
cyanocobalamin, 34
cysteine, 47

dates: cauliflower, banana and date
        salad, 194
    date and fig pudding, 212–13
deodorants, 14
dermatitis, 14, 29
dermis, 4
desserts, 209–22
devilled kidneys, 83–4
devilled poached eggs, 81–2
diet, 30–57
dips, yogurt, 123
dressing, garlic, 100
drink, strawberry yogurt, 76
drugs, 18, 27–30
dry skin, 5, 14, 64
duck: stir-fried duckling with
        mange-tout, 156

eczema, 12, 16, 21, 22, 23, 26, 29, 50,
        54–5, 64–5
eggs: devilled poached eggs, 81–2
    omelette fines herbes, 116
    scrambled eggs with tomato, 84–5
emotional problems, 23–4
environmental problems, 15–17
enzymes, 53–4
epidermis, 3
essential fatty acids (EFAs), 26, 39,
        47–51
evening primrose oil, 50
exercise, 11
exotic fruit salad, 210
eye problems, 65

fair skin, 5
fasting, 56
fennel: stuffed sea trout, 132
    tomato salad with fennel, 185–6
figs: date and fig pudding, 212–13
filo pastry, fish in, 135–6
fish, 125–39
    fish in filo pastry, 135–6
    fish oils, 50, 51
    seafood spaghetti, 113
    see also individual types of fish
flapjacks, sunflower, 230
flowerpot loaves, 235–6
fluid retention, 9, 10, 69
folic acid, 35, 36
freckles, 5
free radicals, 16, 53
fruit, 52, 54
    exotic fruit salad, 210
    fresh fruit platter, 76–7
    fruit compote, 78
    fruit jelly, 211–12
    fruit teabread, 229–30
    see also individual types of fruit

gado gado, 164–5
gamma-linoleic acid (GLA), 48–50
garlic: grated raw vegetables with
        garlic dressing, 100
    potato and garlic purée, 177–8
gazpacho, 96
ginger: date and fig pudding, 212–13
    turkey and ginger stir-fry, 153
goat's cheese tart, 120
golden salad, 192–3

gooseberry and plum tart, 220–21
granary and walnut French sticks,
    233–4
granita, charentais, 216–17
grapes: chicken and grape salad,
    187–8
    grape, watercress and Stilton
        salad, 188
    melon and grape cocktail, 107
Greek-style kebabs, 201
green beans: coriander noodles, 163
    stir-fried green beans with mustard
        seeds, 180
griddle cakes, lemon, 79–80

haddock: haddock and prawn stir-fry,
    134–5
    sweetcorn and haddock chowder,
        97
hake steaks in lime, 202–3
ham: club sandwiches, 236–7
    shredded spinach with smoked ham,
        102–3
hamburgers, 202
hazelnuts: Brussels sprouts with
    hazelnuts, 178
    spinach with raisins and nuts,
        175–6
heartsease, 57
hedgerow salad, 193
herbal remedies, 56–7
herbal teas, 56
herpes, 63
hives, 55
honeyed chicken, 151
hormones, 8–10, 23, 28
horse-tail, 56
hot weather, 15
humidity, 15
hummus, baked jacket potatoes with,
    121
hydrocortisone, 29
hydrolipidic film, 11–12
hydroquinone, 29
hygiene, 14
hyperkeratosis, 31
hypothalamus gland, 22

iatrogenic rosacea, 30
ices: almond and mango ice cream, 218
    apple and lemon sorbet, 215

ices (cont'd)
    charentais granita, 216–17
    raspberry bombe, 217–18
illness, 11
immune system, 11–13, 19, 20, 23, 26,
    30
inositol, 36
iodine, 46
iron, 27, 37, 39, 42–3
isotretinoin, 28

jelly, fruit, 211–12
jetlag, 8

kebabs: chicken and orange, 154
    Greek-style, 201
    marinated lamb, 200
    monkfish and mussels, 203–4
    vegetable, 208
kedgeree, bulgar, 86–7
keratinisation, 3, 31
kidneys: brown rice with kidney and
        bacon, 82–3
    devilled kidneys, 83–4
    sautéed lambs kidneys, 148–9
kippers: bulgar kedgeree, 86–7
    kipper mousse, 104–5
    stir-fried kippers and cucumber,
        115–16

lamb: Greek-style kebabs, 201
    lamb tagine, 143
    marinated lamb kebabs, 200
    rack of lamb in a herb overcoat, 142
langerhans cells, 3
lecithin, 36
leg ulcers, 65
lemon: apple and lemon sorbet, 215
    lemon griddle cakes with
        strawberry sauce, 79–80
lemon sole in lettuce, 128
lentil roulade with mushrooms,
    159–60
lettuce: lemon sole in lettuce, 128
    lettuce and mange-tout soup, 91
light meals, 109–23
lime: hake steaks in lime, 202–3
    sardines with lime and herbs, 133
linoleic acid (LA), 148–50
liver: chicken and orange kebabs, 154
    liver with satsumas, 149–50

liver (cont'd)
    warm chicken liver and bread
        salad, 110
lysine, 47

mackerel: mackerel fillets in oatmeal
        and almonds, 131
    smoked mackerel and new potato
        salad, 138-9
    spiced mackerel, 130
magnesium, 41-2
malignant melanoma, 13, 18
manganese, 43-4
mange-tout: lettuce and mange-tout
        soup, 91
    stir-fried duckling with mange-tout,
        156
mangoes: almond and mango ice
        cream, 218
marigold, 56
marinated lamb kebabs, 200
'mask of pregnancy' (chloasma), 9, 28
meat, 141-50
Mediterranean fish stew, 126
melanin, 3, 5, 17
melon: charentias granita, 216-17
    melon and grape cocktail, 107
menopause, 9
methionine, 47
minerals, 40-42
mint: bass baked in mint, 129
    minted strawberry custards,
        215-16
    smoked chicken and mint salad,
        105-6
moisture, 7-8
monkfish: Mediterranean fish stew,
        126
    monkfish and mussels brochettes,
        203-4
    monkfish in a rich tomato sauce, 127
mousse, kipper, 104-5
muesli: crumbly muesli bars, 231
    mixed nut and seed muesli, 79
muffins, spiced oatmeal, 77-8
mullet, barbecued, 205
mushrooms: aubergine and bean
        gratin, 119-20
    devilled poached eggs, 81-2
    lentil roulade with mushrooms,
        159-60

mushrooms (cont'd)
    mushroom and cashew toasts, 85-6
    mushroom soufflé, 117
    steamed greens with mushrooms,
        179
mussels: Mediterranean fish stew,
        126
    monkfish and mussels
        brochettes, 203-4
    mussels in tomato sauce, 114-15
    seafood spaghetti, 113
mustard: mustard chicken drumsticks,
        204-5
    stir-fried green beans with mustard
        seeds, 180

nectarine, cold spiced pork with, 146
nerves, 4
niacin, 33-4
noodles, coriander, 163
nutrition, 30-57
nuts: mixed grain and nut salad, 197-8
    mixed nut and seed muesli, 79
    nut and cheese plait, 166-7
    nut soda bread, 80-81

oatmeal: apricot oat crunchies, 227-8
    mackerel fillets in oatmeal and
        almonds, 131
    roasted oatmeal vegetables, 176-7
    spiced oatmeal muffins, 77-8
    sunflower flapjacks, 230
oedema, 69-70
oestrogens, 8-10, 28
oily skin, 5, 14, 18, 66
olives: goat's cheese tarts, 120
omelette fines herbes, 116
onions: roasted oatmeal vegetables,
        176-7
orange: apricot and orange soufflés,
        213-14
    asparagus with orange sauce,
        100-101
    chicken and orange kebabs, 154
    fruit jelly, 211-12
Oriental salad, 191-2
Oriental skin, 5-6, 20
osmotic oedema, 10
osteomalacia, 20
osteoporosis, 9
oxidation, 15-16, 24, 39, 53, 54

ozone layer, 20

PABA (para-amino-benzoic-acid), 36
pallor, 66–7
pantothenic acid, 35–6
parsnips: roasted oatmeal vegetables,
    176–7
passion fruit: strawberry and passion
    fruit Swiss roll, 228–9
pasta shells with cheese and walnuts,
    164
peaches, raspberry chicken with,
    150–51
peanut cookies, 232–3
pears: pear and nut cake, 224–5
    pears with blackcurrant sauce, 211
    red cabbage with pears, 184
    walnut pear slice, 219
pellagra, 33
peppers: courgette and pepper salad,
    190
    gazpacho, 96
    pepper salad, 189
    spicy black beans and rice, 158
    turkey and ginger stir-fry, 153
phosphorus, 40–41
pie, ratatouille cheese, 167–8
pigmentation, 39
pineapple: golden salad, 192–3
    haddock and prawn stir-fry, 134–5
pituitary gland, 21
plums: gooseberry and plum tart,
    220–21
PMT (pre-menstrual tension), 9
pollution, 13–14, 16, 24
pork: apricot and redcurrant stuffed
    pork, 147–8
    cold spiced pork with nectarine, 146
potassium, 41
potato: baked jacket potatoes with
    hummus, 121
    potato and garlic purée, 177–8
    smoked mackerel and new potato
        salad, 138–9
    spinach and cheese quiche with
        crisp potato crust, 118
poultry, 150–56
prawns: haddock and prawn stir-fry
    134–5
    Mediterranean fish stew, 126
    mixed seafood salad, 137–8
    prawn risotto, 111

pregnancy, 9
progestogen, 28
prostaglandins, 48–50
prunes: fruit jelly, 211–12
psoriasis, 13, 16, 22, 23, 27, 29, 31,
    38, 51, 55, 67
psychotherapy, 23–4
puddings, 209–22
pyridoxine, 34

quiches see tarts

rack of lamb in a herb overcoat, 142
raisins: spinach with raisins and nuts,
    175–6
raspberries: raspberry bombe, 217–18
    raspberry chicken with peaches,
        150–51
ratatouille cheese pie, 167–8
raw foods, 52–4
red cabbage with pears, 184
red cherry soup, 95
red kidney beans: bean, cheese and
    avocado salad, 196
    bean and chicken tabouleh, 112
red mullet, barbecued 205
redcurrants: apricot and redcurrant
    stuffed pork, 147–8
retinoic acid, 28, 32
retinol see vitamin A
rhubarb brown Betty, 220
riboflavin, 33
rice: brown rice with kidney and
    bacon, 82–3
    mixed grain and nut salad, 197–8
    prawn risotto, 111
    spicy black beans and rice, 158
    vegetable risotto, 160–61
rickets, 20
risottos: prawn, 111
    vegetable, 160–61
roulade, lentil with mushrooms, 159–60

St John's wort, 57
salads, 183–98
    avocado and chick-peas, 122
    bean, cheese and avocado, 196
    cauliflower, banana and date, 194
    celeriac, 186–7
    chicken and grape, 187–8
    courgette and pepper, 190
    crunchy winter salad, 184–5

salads (cont'd)
  curried apple coleslaw, 190–91
  gado gado, 164–5
  Golden salad, 192–3
  grape, watercress and Stilton, 188
  hedgerow, 193
  mixed grain and nut, 197–8
  mixed seafood, 137–8
  Oriental, 191–2
  pepper, 189
  red cabbage with pears, 184
  salade Niçoise, 136–7
  smoked chicken and mint, 105–6
  smoked mackerel and new potato, 138–9
  sprouted, 195
  tomato with fennel, 185–6
  warm chicken liver and bread, 110
  warm whitebait, 106
sallowness, 66
salt, 41
sandwiches, club, 236–7
sardines with lime and herbs, 133
satsumas, liver with, 149–50
sauces: blackcurrant, 211
  orange, 100–101
  rich tomato, 127
  strawberry, 79–80
  tomato, 114, 170, 174
scallops: mixed seafood salad, 137–8
sea trout, stuffed, 132
seafood spaghetti, 113
sebaceous glands, 10
seborrheic dermatitis, 9
sebum, 4
seeds: mixed nut and seed muesli, 79
selenium, 16, 39, 44
sesame seed biscuits, 232
'stick office' skin, 16–17
silicon, 44
skin: nutrition, 30–57
  problems, 6–30, 59–71
  structure and function, 2–4
  types, 5–6
smoked chicken and mint salad, 105–6
smoked mackerel and new potato salad, 138–9
smoking, 8, 15, 23, 24–5
snacks, 109–23
soap, 14
soap-wort, 56

soda bread, 80–81
sodium, 41
sole: lemon sole in lettuce, 128
sorbet, apple and lemon, 215
soufflés: apricot and orange, 213–14
  mushroom, 117
soups: avocado, 94
  cold cucumber, 93–4
  gazpacho, 96
  lettuce and mange-tout, 91
  red cherry, 95
  spinach, 91–2
  sweetcorn and haddock chowder, 97
  watercress, 92–3
  winter vegetable, 90
spaghetti, seafood, 113
spiced fruit cake, 225–6
spiced mackerel, 130
spiced oatmeal muffins, 77–8
spicy apple cake, 224
spicy black beans and rice, 158
spinach: avocado and chick-peas salad, 122
  shredded spinach with smoked ham, 102–3
  spinach and cheese quiche with crisp potato crust, 118–19
  spinach with raisins and nuts, 175–6
  spinach soup, 91–2
spring greens, steamed with mushrooms, 179
sprouted salad, 195
squid: Mediterranean fish stew, 126
starters, 99–107
stews: beef Burgundy, 144
  lamb tagine, 143
  Mediterranean fish stew, 126
Stilton, grape and watercress salad, 188
stinging nettles, 56
strawberries: lemon griddle cakes with strawberry sauce, 79–80
  minted strawberry custards, 215–16
  strawberry and passion fruit Swiss roll, 228–9
  strawberry yogurt drink, 76
stress, 13, 21–3, 26
stretch marks, 68
sulphur, 45
sunburn, 17, 19, 68–9

sunflower flapjacks, 230
sunlight, 17–18
sweat glands, 4, 7, 12
sweetcorn and haddock chowder, 97
swelling, 69–70

tabouleh, bean and chicken, 112
tagliatelle: coriander noodles, 163
tagine, lamb, 143
tandoori chicken, 206
tarts: basil and tomato tartlets, 101–2
    goat's cheese tarts, 120
    gooseberry and plum tart, 220–21
    spinach and cheese quiche with
        crisp potato crust, 118–19
tea, 23, 26–7, 43
teabreads: cottage cheese and Brazil
        nut teabread, 226–7
    fruit teabread, 229–30
testosterone, 23, 28
thiamin, 33
Thousand Island dip, 123
thrush, 70–71
thyroid gland, 10
tofu: almond and mango ice cream,
    218
tomato: basil and tomato tartlets,
        101–2
    celeriac with tomato sauce, 174
    chicken Parmigiana, 152
    curried fish with coconut, 133–4
    devilled poached eggs, 81–2
    gazpacho, 96
    monkfish in a rich tomato sauce, 127
    mussels in tomato sauce, 114–15
    ratatouille cheese pie, 167–8
    scrambled eggs with tomato, 84–5
    tomato salad with fennel, 185–6
    vegetable loaf with tomato sauce,
        170–71
trace elements, 42–6, 52
tuna: salade Niçoise, 136–7
turkey: club sandwiches, 236–7
    turkey and ginger stir-fry, 153
tyrosine, 47

ulcers, leg, 65
ultraviolet light, 17–19, 38

VDUs, 16
vegetables, 52, 54
    accompanying dishes, 173–81

vegetables (cont'd)
    grated raw vegetables with garlic
        dressing, 100
    vegetable curry, 162
    vegetable kebabs, 208
    vegetable loaf with tomato sauce,
        170–71
    vegetable risotto, 160–61
    yogurt dips with crudités, 123
    see also individual types of
        vegetables and salads
vegetarian dishes, 157–71
veins, broken, 5, 26, 61–2
virus infections, 12
vitamin A, 16, 28, 30, 31, 38, 39, 50
vitamin B complex, 23, 25, 27, 32–7,
    43, 45, 52
vitamin C, 16, 23, 25, 27, 30, 37–8, 39,
    43, 52
vitamin D, 20–21, 31, 38, 40, 50
vitamin E, 16, 31, 39–40, 44, 51
vitamin F see essential fatty acids
vitamin K, 31
vitiligo, 13, 23

walnuts: granary and walnut French
        sticks, 233–4
    pasta shells with cheese and
        walnuts, 164
    pear and nut cake, 224–5
    walnut pear slice, 219
warm chicken liver and bread salad,
    110
water chestnuts: haddock and prawn
        stir-fry, 134–5
    stir-fried duckling with mange-tout,
        156
watercress: grape, watercress and
        Stilton salad, 188
    watercress soup, 92–3
Wheat: mixed grain and nut salad,
    197–8
whitebait salad, 106
winter vegetable soup, 90
wounds, 71

yogurt: spiced mackerel, 130
    strawberry yogurt drink, 176
    yogurt dips with crudités, 123

zinc, 23, 27, 30, 31, 40, 43, 45–6

More Cookery Non-Fiction from Headline:

GOOD HOUSEKEEPING

GOOD FOOD
FOR
Diabetics

THEODORA FITZGIBBON

GOOD HOUSEKEEPING
— the recipe for healthy living

At last: a cookbook for diabetics with recipes that are so delicious that *all* the family will want to eat them.

Drawing on her own personal experience of diabetes coupled with her vast professional knowledge, Theodora FitzGibbon, author of over 30 cookbooks and longstanding cookery editor of the *Irish Times,* has specially created over 150 recipes suitable for diabetics, each with its own at-a-glance chart giving carbohydrate, fibre and energy values. With recipes for everything from quick meals (Gratin of Eggs) to special occasions (Paupiette de Boeuf), well-informed general advice on the diabetic diet and a comprehensive list of raw ingredients and their food values, *Good Food for Diabetics* is a priceless addition to the kitchens of all diabetics and their families.

'Overall, a good book to buy' *Balance,* official magazine of the British Diabetic Association

'No cookery reference shelf would be complete without a collection of the books of that great cook, Theodora FitzGibbon' *Sunday Telegraph*

NON-FICTION/COOKERY   0 7472 3280 6   £4.99

GUY SAVOY WITH GUY LANGLOIS

VEGETABLE

MAGIC

"ONE OF THE MOST IMAGINATIVE CHEFS OF HIS GENERATION."
CHRISTIAN MILLAU

"The dish is not born in the kitchen. I think of it, I imagine it and when it's ripe in my head, I make it."

Recognised as one of the most talented young chefs of his generation, Guy Savoy served his apprenticeship with the Troisgros brothers before opening his two Paris restaurants, which now command 3 toques and 18/20 in the Gault-Millau guide.

Taking vegetables as the focal point and using ingredients that are familiar to every cook, Guy Savoy creates exquisite first courses, side dishes and main courses by subtle balancing and mingling of tastes and textures. His delicious combinations include cauliflower with watercress purée, lobster with asparagus mousse and carpaccio of duck with chicory.

Guy Savoy's remarkable talent for harmonising foods takes vegetables to new heights, producing exquisite and original tastes with everyday ingredients. It's sheer magic!

"A rising young giant of French cuisine." *A La Carte*

NON-FICTION/FOOD AND WINE   0 7472 3161 3   £5.99

A selection of bestsellers
from Headline

FICTION

TALENT	Nigel Rees	£3.99 ☐
A BLOODY FIELD BY SHREWSBURY	Edith Pargeter	£3.99 ☐
GUESTS OF THE EMPEROR	Janice Young Brooks	£3.99 ☐
THE LAND IS BRIGHT	Elizabeth Murphy	£3.99 ☐
THE FACE OF FEAR	Dean R Koontz	£3.50 ☐

NON-FICTION

CHILD STAR	Shirley Temple Black	£4.99 ☐
BLIND IN ONE EAR	Patrick Macnee and Marie Cameron	£3.99 ☐
TWICE LUCKY	John Francome	£4.99 ☐
HEARTS AND SHOWERS	Su Pollard	£2.99 ☐

SCIENCE FICTION AND FANTASY

WITH FATE CONSPIRE The Destiny Makers 1	Mike Shupp	£3.99 ☐
A DISAGREEMENT WITH DEATH	Craig Shaw Gardner	£2.99 ☐
SWORD & SORCERESS 4	Marion Zimmer Bradley	£3.50 ☐

All Headline books are available at your local bookshop or newsagent, or can be ordered direct from the publisher. Just tick the titles you want and fill in the form below. Prices and availability subject to change without notice.

Headline Book Publishing PLC, Cash Sales Department, PO Box 11, Falmouth, Cornwall TR10 9EN, England.

Please enclose a cheque or postal order to the value of the cover price and allow the following for postage and packing:
UK: 60p for the first book, 25p for the second book and 15p for each additional book ordered up to a maximum charge of £1.90
BFPO: 60p for the first book, 25p for the second book and 15p per copy for the next seven books, thereafter 9p per book
OVERSEAS & EIRE: £1.25 for the first book, 75p for the second book and 28p for each subsequent book.

Name ....

Address ....

....

....